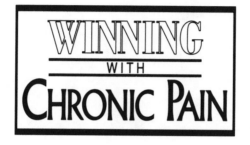

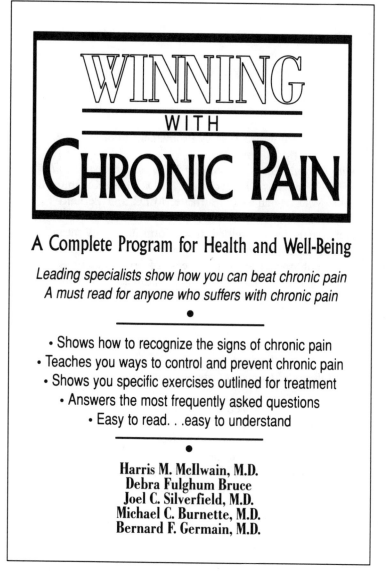

WINNING
WITH
CHRONIC PAIN

A Complete Program for Health and Well-Being

Leading specialists show how you can beat chronic pain
A must read for anyone who suffers with chronic pain

•

- Shows how to recognize the signs of chronic pain
- Teaches you ways to control and prevent chronic pain
- Shows you specific exercises outlined for treatment
- Answers the most frequently asked questions
- Easy to read. . .easy to understand

•

Harris M. McIlwain, M.D.
Debra Fulghum Bruce
Joel C. Silverfield, M.D.
Michael C. Burnette, M.D.
Bernard F. Germain, M.D.

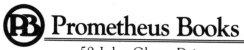 **Prometheus Books**

59 John Glenn Drive
Amherst, New York 14228-2197

Published 1994 by Prometheus Books

98 97 96 95 94   5 4 3 2 1

Library of Congress Cataloging-in-Publication Data

Winning with chronic pain : a complete program for health and well-being /
    Harris H. McIlwain . . . [et al.].
        p.   cm. — (Consumer health library)
    Includes bibliographical references.
    ISBN 0-87975-900-3 (cloth) — ISBN 0-87975-878-3 (paper)
    1. Chronic pain—Popular works. I. McIlwain, Harris H. II. Series.
RB127.W55   1994
616'.0472—dc20   94-2443
                                                                          CIP

Printed in the United States of America on acid-free paper.

In honor of our beloved grandmother,
Nina Ellis Holden,
born September 29, 1895.

In celebration of her life, good health and
positive outlook on life.

Contents

List of Trademark Medications

Advil is a trademark of Whitehall Laboratories, Inc.

Anacin 3 is a trademark of Whitehall Laboratories, Inc.

Anaprox is a trademark for Syntex Laboratories, Inc.

Ansaid is a tradename of the Upjohn Company

Aristocort is a trademark of Lederle Laboratories, a division of American Cynamid Company

Arthritis Strength Ascriptin is a trademark of Rorer Consumer Pharmaceuticals

Arthritis Strength Tri-Buffered Bufferin is a trademark of Bristol-Meyers Products

Ascriptin is a trademark of Rorer Consumer Pharmaceuticals

Ascriptin A/D is a trademark of Rorer Consumer Pharmaceuticals

Bayer Aspirin is a trademark of Glenbrook Laboratories

Biocal is a trademark of Miles, Inc., Consumer Healthcare Division

Calcet is a trademark of Mission Pharmaceutical Company

Clinoril is a trademark of Merck, Sharpe & Dohme, a division of Merck & Co., Inc.

Darvon is a trademark of Eli Lilly Company

Daypro is a trademark of G. D. Searle & Co.

Decadron is a trademark of Merck, Sharpe & Dohme, a division of Merck & Co., Inc.

Deltasone is a trademark of the Upjohn Company

Depen is a trademark of Wallace Laboratories

Digel is a trademark of Shering-Plough Health Care

Disalcid is a trademark of 3M Riker

Dorcal is a trademark of Sandoz Consumer Health Care Group Division of Sandoz, Inc.

Easprin is a trademark of Parke-Davis

Eight-Hour Bayer Timed Release is a trademark of Glenbrook Laboratories

Elavil is a trademark of Merck, Sharpe & Dohme, a division of Merck & Co., Inc.

Emperin is a trademark of Burroughs-Wellcome Company

Flexeril is a trademark of Merck, Sharpe & Dohme, a division of Merck & Co., Inc.

Imuran is a trademark of Burroughs-Wellcome Company

Indocin is a trademark of Merck, Sharpe & Dohme, a division of Merck & Co., Inc.

Lorcet is a trademark of VAD Laboratories

Lortab is a trademark of Russ Pharmaceuticals, Inc.

Meclomen is a trademark of Parke-Davis

Medrol is a trademark of the Upjohn Company

Metacortin is a trademark of Schering Corporation

Myochrisine is a trademark of Merck, Sharpe & Dohme, a division of Merck & Co., Inc.

Nalfon is a trademark of Dista Products Company, a division of Eli Lilly Company

Orasone is a trademark of Reider Rowell

Orudis is a trademark of Winthrop Pharmaceuticals

Panadol is a trademark of Glenbrook Laboratories

Parafon Forte is a trademark of McNeil Pharmaceuticals

Paxil is a trademark of Smith Line Laboratories

Percocet is a trademark of DuPont Pharmaceuticals

Phenaphen with Codeine is a trademark of A.H. Robbins Company, Inc.

Plaquenil is a trademark of Winthrop Pharmaceuticals

Rheumatrex is a trademark of Lederle Laboratories

Ridaura is a trademark of Smith, Kline and French

Robaxin is a trademark of A.H. Robbins Company, Inc.

Salflex is a trademark of Carnrick Laboratories, Inc.

Sinequan is a trademark of Roerig Division, Pfizer, Inc.

Skelaxin is a trademark of Carnrick Laboratories, Inc.

Solgonal is a trademark of Schering Corporation

Soma is a trademark of Wallace Laboratories

Talacen is a trademark of Winthrop Pharmaceuticals

Talwin is trademark of Winthrop Pharmaceuticals

Titralac is a trademark of 3M Corporation

Tofranil is a trademark of Geigy Pharmaceuticals

Tolectin is a trademark of McNeil Pharmaceuticals

Trilisate is a trademark of The Purdue Frederick Company

Tums is a trademark of Norcliff Thayer, Inc.

Tylenol is a trademark of McNeil Pharmaceuticals

Tylox is a trademark of McNeil Pharmaceuticals

Valium is a trademark of Roche Laboratories

Introduction

Have you ever had a throbbing headache—one that would not quit and continued all day and into the night? Imagine having this same headache every waking moment to the point where it is all you think about. Envision that everywhere you go throughout the day, your head throbs, pulsates, and sends painful messages throughout your body—and that nothing seems to help.

What about a sharp pain in your back? Have you ever injured your back and experienced a piercing pain for a day or two? Imagine having this same penetrating pain every day and every night for weeks and months; no matter what you do to alleviate this pain, it is still there keeping you from sleeping or working.

More than 100 million people suffer from chronic pain every day and experience this excruciating agony every waking moment. They lose sleep each night to this constant reminder of back pain, arthritis pain, headache pain, neck pain, nerve pain, the pain of cancer or other diseases, and experience inactivity during daytime hours. Most people with chronic pain, after going from physician to physician for treatment or cures, often give up hope of ever having a normal life. This resignation leads to feelings of depression, anxiety, and hopelessness.

But this does not have to be—there is hope for people with chronic pain! While it may be that the pain cannot be totally erased, it is possible for sufferers to begin a treatment plan so that they can live a meaningful, normal life, focusing on the very things that are important: relationships with family and friends, work, community activities, travel, and more.

Each day in our clinic we treat people with chronic pain, and we know that help is available, *if* our patients are willing to follow a method of treatment directed at that specific pain. In *Winning with Chronic Pain,* we have targeted the most common causes of chronic pain and explained the modes of treatment prescribed. We also offer important case studies of patients who are winning with chronic pain right now, and an entire chapter is devoted to answering the questions most people have regarding their pain and the available treatment programs.

It is important to understand that you don't have to suffer alone any more. If you have chronic pain, you can feel comfort knowing that you are *not* alone. For all who suffer with chronic pain: once a diagnosis is made, there *is* hope for treatment.

Winning with chronic pain is a possibility for the 100 million sufferers in America today. But it is up to you to make the effort to understand the cause of your pain; begin a treatment plan specifically designed for this type of pain; exercise daily; control your stress; and, if needed, seek new modes of treatment. Then you will be on the road to recovery.

For those who read this book, it is our desire that lives will be changed as new insights are given in how to manage chronic pain.

We greatly appreciate the contributions from these professionals who donated time and talents to make *Winning with Chronic Pain* complete: Francis I. Barford, L.O.T.R.; Dana S. Deboskey, Ph.D.; Susan Haley, R.D., L.D.; Daniel McIlwain; Virginia McIlwain; Michael McIlwain; Dominador U. Martirez, R.P.T., L.P.T.; Suni Petersen, M.A., L.M.H.C. (president of The Mind-Body Connection); Stephen F. Russell, Ph.D.; Gordon S. Saskin, M.D.; Vernon L. Swenson, Ph.D.; St. Joseph's Hospital Medical Library, Tampa, Florida; Tampa Medical Group, P.A.; Vicki K. Windsor, R.P.T.; and Gary L. Wood, Ph.D.

1

Start Winning Today with Chronic Pain

If you are reading this book, the chances are great that you or someone you know is suffering with chronic pain. This unending misery may be the result of excruciating back pain, a debilitating injury, the constant pain of arthritis or headache, nerve pain, or the pain of cancer. While chronic pain does restrict the lives of more than 100 million people each year, living with it does not have to be an ordeal. You *can* win the battle with chronic pain.

Winning with Chronic Pain was written to offer new hope to the millions who suffer from interminable pain. In this book we will tell you how people from all around the world are now living busy and normal lives—even with their chronic pain. We will give you examples of the most common types of chronic pain and let you know ways to treat this pain *today*. This book will explain the importance of exercise and movement to *end* pain, tell when surgery might be an option, and show you how to manage your weight and your stress. It will teach you how to prevent more pain as you become active and begin to enjoy a fuller life.

Following are some excellent examples of what we mean.

Janet C. suffers from chronic pain. Not only did Janet win Teacher of the Year award in her small southern community last June, she is now running for the school board. Janet's enthusiasm is contagious—from the way she handles her class to her involvement with the after school club she sponsors, even to the way she walks in the evenings with her husband. To watch Janet as she actively tackles each day, one would never guess that she is in constant pain.

Yet seven years ago, a car accident left Janet with chronic back pain due to a herniated disc. After going from physician to therapist, spending thousands of dollars and hours on cures and relief, then having lengthy surgery with unfavorable results, Janet has finally learned how to control her pain with the same steps described in this book. While her physical pain has not completely ended, she is able to live a normal, active life and do the things she wants without debilitating pain holding her back.

William Z. is another active person who is winning with chronic pain. A job-related accident left him with a severe neck injury, and William nearly became an invalid as he stayed in bed day and night, trying to escape his pain.

"When I finally realized that my pain was not going to leave until I addressed my total being, I found relief," William said. "I have learned that everything I do each day and how I react to these stresses mentally, emotionally, and physically, all contribute to my pain."

William also learned some tips on winning with chronic neck pain as he followed the program outlined in this book.

If you suffer with constant long-lasting pain (chronic pain), you know the sacrifices William and Janet have confronted: loss of employment, loss of time at work, and the loss of money as they sought ways to relieve the pain. Other problems, including broken relationships with family and friends, depression, and losing the will to live, have faced William and Janet and millions of other people who live with chronic pain.

MORE THAN 100 MILLION PEOPLE HAVE CHRONIC PAIN

If you have chronic pain, you are not alone. Some researchers estimate that as many as one third of all Americans at some time suffer from some type of chronic pain. This means that more than 100 million people have shared the same problem with you. Yes, there are over 37 million Americans with arthritis, 32 million with chronic back pain, over 30 million with chronic headaches, and over 15 million who suffer with the constant pain of cancer and other illnesses that create painful disabilities. Did you know that chronic back pain is the most common disability in people under age forty-five?

1. Number of people
with various types of chronic pain

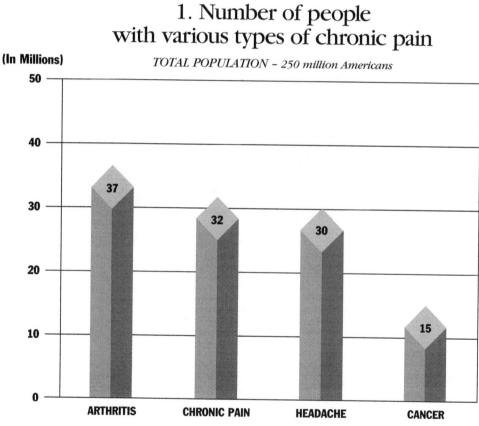

Table 1.1. Number of persons suffering with chronic pain

PERSONS SUFFERING WITH CHRONIC PAIN

It is so easy to feel lost, overwhelmed, and beaten by chronic pain. This is not hard to understand when you consider what chronic pain can do. It greets you as you awaken in the morning. It reminds you of its existence throughout the day, holding you back from performing the very activities that are normal and necessary, including going to work or enjoying your family. Chronic pain is still there as you prepare for bed; its nagging signals interrupt your sleep. As you have probably already experienced, chronic pain can change people who are normally happy and free into miserable and limited individuals.

CHRONIC PAIN IS *NOT* IN YOUR HEAD

If you have chronic pain, well-meaning friends and family members have probably offered one or more of the following observations:

- If you don't think about it, it will go away.
- Since the medication isn't working, perhaps it is in your head.
- You don't look like you're in pain. Are you sure it isn't something else?
- Just put the pain out of your mind.
- Maybe if you move around more, the pain will go away.
- You always did have a vivid imagination.
- Maybe you should stop taking that medication. It probably isn't helping.

After suffering with endless, piercing pain day after day, year after year, you may even start to think that perhaps you are fabricating the pain or that maybe the pain really is "in your head."

Chronic pain is *not* in your head; it is very real. While your emotions can and will affect the amount of pain you might feel, the pain itself is genuine.

THE COSTS OF CHRONIC PAIN

In addition to the cost in suffering each year to the millions of persons with chronic pain, the financial expense can be devastating. For example, in chronic back pain there are healthcare and medication costs. These could be many thousands of dollars, not including the costs of specialized tests, hospitalization, or surgery.

After an extended length of treatment with little control of pain and more loss of activity, a person suffering from chronic pain, such as back pain, may be referred to a pain clinic. An inpatient pain clinic with a four- to six-week program can be a very good form of treatment, but this alone may cost $20,000 or more.

While 40 to 60 percent of patients have a good response to an intensive pain center evaluation and treatment, there are many others who continue to suffer even after such a large expenditure of health care funds.

It is difficult to estimate the actual dollar cost that the average chronic pain sufferer incurs. It is estimated that over 700 million work days are lost each year to chronic pain, accounting for a large amount of the total loss of work.

With ongoing healthcare, loss of income, and other expenses, the cost to the nation of chronic back pain alone has been estimated to be anywhere from $50 billion to $75 billion each year. This does not begin to include the expense due to arthritis pain, chronic headaches, and other chronic pain.

Added to this expense is the human cost of suffering to both patient and family as a result of chronic pain. This will be discussed in later chapters.

The good news is that large savings in healthcare costs are possible if only a small percentage of improvement in chronic pain could be achieved. And the improvement in human costs could affect millions of people.

FROM PATIENT TO PERSON

For those who suffer with chronic pain there is hope. The pain can be controlled, and you can begin to live a normal life. Of course, the best hope is to get rid of the pain by removing the cause or finding a treatment that eliminates the pain altogether. But in many cases, that simply cannot be done because the cures for many causes of chronic pain have not been discovered.

But it is now known that most of those who suffer from chronic pain can get relief. They don't have simply to live with the pain anymore, and they can begin to live a normal life, engaging in the activities they enjoy.

The main ingredient in the treatment of chronic pain is *you*. Even if the pain may never completely go away, *if* you begin a comprehensive program, including exercise, moist heat, stress control, medication, and more, the chronic pain that once agonized you can become tolerable.

In other words, you can change things so that you get around and do the things you want to do in reasonable comfort, without severe limitation by the pain. You can begin to live your life again and move from patient to person—from happier times at home to improved quality times at work and play.

MANAGING YOUR CHRONIC PAIN

You can learn to manage pain just as you manage other areas of your life. We will show you how to gain control over the pain and your life. Of course, the ultimate goal is to eliminate the pain. But if this is not possible, then you can learn to manage it rather than letting the pain take control. There are enough available ways to treat chronic pain, so that most persons can now expect to experience relief.

Martha W. is a fifty-five-year-old woman who has had severe back pain for three years. She suffered from arthritis of the spine and had several fractures in the bones of the spine from thinning of the bones (osteoporosis). The severe pain caused Martha to become stooped over and to experience trouble walking. She could not sleep well at night and was always tired in the morning.

"I honestly thought that my body had totally failed me," Martha said. "I could no longer go to church or on family outings with my grandchildren, and I was afraid to hug anyone for fear of pain. The pain had absolutely ruined my life."

When Martha had proper diagnosis of the causes of her pain, she started immediate treatment for each cause. After six months, Martha became a different person! She was able to walk a mile, sleep through the night without awakening from pain, and she finally felt that the pain no longer limited her. Martha began to control her pain rather than let it take over her life. She last reported that she was going on a two-week vacation with her grandchildren.

Sandy R., a forty-year-old woman, works as a legal secretary. She suffered from chronic headaches and such intense jaw pain that she frequently was unable to go to work. After enduring for several years, Sandy had missed work so often that she expected to lose her job.

"The jaw pain was horrible, leaving my entire neck, ears, and head rigid with pain almost every day," Sandy said. "The pain affected my moods and my relationships with family members and co-workers."

After testing, she was found to have a common cause of chronic headaches and neck pain. With treatment, including daily medication, moist heat and stress reduction, Sandy now controls the pain. While she still has some headaches and some jaw pain, she is now in control. Since learning how to manage her chronic pain, Sandy excels in her work and recently received a raise in salary. She has resumed her active social life and has shifted from being a patient to being a person.

Reginald J., fifty years old, had a problem with pain in his legs. The pain was sharp and burning and was felt through both legs below the knees. This pain was especially bothersome at night, so much so that Reginald would often awaken. For several years he ignored the pain during the day while he was active, but the pain at night was so limiting that he dreaded going to bed.

Reginald was found to have pain caused by the nerves in his legs reacting to another medical problem. The underlying medical problem was treated, and medication was given at night to treat the nerve pain. He now has relief of the nighttime leg pain. This has allowed him to sleep without interruption and to feel rested each morning. Reginald feels better overall, and he is not as tired during the day.

TRY A MULTIDISCIPLINARY APPROACH

If you have chronic pain, like thousands of other sufferers, you have probably tried many ways to obtain relief—biofeedback, medications, surgery, and counseling. But to control the pain, you may need to take a multidisciplinary approach that involves several measures for relief.

Treat yourself as a whole person. This book will outline a program that can help you do just that.

TAKE RESPONSIBILITY FOR YOUR PAIN

Jack S. suffered with arthritis in his knees for years. When the pain became so unbearable that he had to stop working, he knew he had to find treatment.

"I always thought that medication would give me enough relief to get through the day," Jack said. "When the medication stopped working, and I had to leave my job, I was frightened. I didn't know where to turn."

After Jack began a multidisciplinary program, like the one outlined in this book—including moist heat, medications, exercise, and stress management—he could begin work again.

"I have learned that it is all right to have limitations, and now I take one day at a time. The pain is controlled if I stay on my treatment, and it is my responsibility to take this control."

Another sufferer with chronic headache pain, Laura B., had no difficulty believing that her headaches always intensified after a stressful day at her law office. "After a day of meetings or being in court, I could always count on an evening of lying in bed with a tension headache," she said. "The pain is so unbearable, and usually after it comes on, the medication doesn't even help.

"But what finally helped me was learning to handle those situations that added to my stress. I have now learned that some biofeedback techniques, along with my medication, help me control my chronic pain. I have to be in charge of this pain, and now I'm winning."

RELIEF IS AVAILABLE

As you read this book and use the methods described to eliminate or relieve your pain, remember that you have lived with chronic pain for a long time—only time and care will overcome it. But many people with chronic pain can find reasonable relief quickly using the various methods we describe. For others, it may take more time, but if you are determined to relieve your pain and work hard with the multidisciplinary approach, you *can* win.

2

Do You Have Chronic Pain?

Chronic pain is long-lasting, often intense pain. Researchers consider pain that lasts from one to six months longer than expected to be chronic, but this time can vary depending on the problem that causes the pain. For example, if a back injury causes acute pain, that is no better after three months, then it is called chronic back pain. Also, pain that returns again and again for months or years can be considered chronic. For example, headaches that are severe and recur many times over one or more years are chronic in nature.

ACUTE PAIN

Acute pain is important because it brings to our attention a problem that is causing or might cause damage to the body. Acute pain could be a toothache from a cavity, a broken bone, a headache from a sinus infection, or a backache from a strain. Muscle pains, joint pain, and pain in the stomach could all be acute signals to warn us of a potential problem. Some injuries can cause acute pain such as bursitis pain from working in the yard at home or tendinitis from playing tennis. Each of these types of acute pain "runs its course" and disappears as the problem is relieved.

Surveys have shown that over 70 percent of Americans have acute pain from headache at some time each year, and over 50 percent of Americans experience backaches on a more regular basis. These pains usually last from a few days to several weeks. When the problem is relieved or the injury heals, then the pain subsides. For example, acute back pain is so common that most adults in America experience it at some time in their lives. In fact, except for the common cold, it is the most common cause of loss of work. Acute back pain can come on suddenly and can be severe, but in over 80 percent of cases it goes away in about two weeks.

Chronic pain occurs when the acute pain lasts far longer than would be expected from the apparent problem. When acute back pain continues for more than a couple of weeks and on into months, then it is considered *chronic back pain.*

CHRONIC PAIN IS DIFFERENT

When the pain becomes chronic, our bodies begin to behave differently. The pain causes the sufferer to awaken repeatedly every night. This results in poor sleep, poor rest, and in the morning, waking up feeling too tired to start the day. Interruptions in sleep at night may create problems of drowsiness during the daytime.

Continued pain causes more irritation and difficulty dealing with others, including family members, friends, and people at work.

THE STAGES OF CHRONIC PAIN

Some researchers have found that many persons who suffer with chronic pain go through several stages or phases.* Early on, there is medical treatment, loss of work, good support from the family, and sometimes surgery to treat the pain. After a few months the limitation of activity causes loss of quality in the person's social and family life. It may then be realized that surgery or other treatment will not cure the pain. Feelings of anger and disappointment grow. The use of narcotics, alcohol, or other drugs may increase as the person in pain tries to get relief.

As time goes on, there is increased loss of activity, and there may be heavy use of narcotics and alcohol. These strong medications, used to control the pain, are usually not very effective, and they can become habit-forming. The sufferer may have less appetite and may lose weight. Or sometimes the stress of chronic pain may cause excessive eating and weight gain.

Problems with family relationships usually increase. The stress of dealing with pain can make everyone in the family more tense and irritable. The person in pain may see many doctors in an effort to find

---

*Fisher et al., *The Clinical Journal of Pain* 1990, 6:191–98.

relief, but with each failed attempt there is less and less hope that something will actually work to relieve the pain.

THE CYCLE OF CHRONIC PAIN

People who suffer with chronic pain often are depressed and withdrawn, so much so that they spend more time away from other people. They can become ever more focused on their pain and suffering, which is very real. The many appointments with healthcare providers to try to find relief, combined with the cost of these attempts, add to the frustration of chronic pain.

As time goes on, those who suffer with pain can have trouble keeping a job: the absences become too frequent. If income is reduced or lost altogether, this adds to the financial stress for the victims of pain and their families. The stress of dealing with loss of income *and* chronic pain can cause severe relationship problems in the family. The rate of divorce is higher in such families.

The longer the same pain situation lasts, the more likely the person will experience feelings and notice signs caused by the stress, including:

- constant fatigue

- lack of interest in other activities

- difficulty concentrating

- increased irritability

- withdrawal from other activities (especially enjoyable ones)

- changes in appetite

- depression.

Each of us shows stress in different ways. It is important for each of us to try to understand the ways in which we show stress that comes with prolonged pain. Then we can begin taking steps to control the stress. The problems associated with managing stress and chronic pain are discussed in chapter 7.

The goal is to reach the stage at which chronic pain can be controlled. Each of us can learn to live with our pain *without* narcotics. Once this is accomplished, returning to work is a possibility, as are improved sleep and no limitations caused by depression.

LOOKING AT THE FACTS

It is estimated that over one third of all Americans may suffer from chronic pain at some time, and that one in six of us suffers from pain at any given time. Let's look at some of the most common causes of chronic pain, including back pain, arthritis, and headaches. Also important are jaw and face pain, neck pain, cancer pain, and nerve pain.

CHRONIC BACK PAIN

Chronic back pain cripples over 2.5 million Americans each year. This pain can affect any part of the back, but the *lower* (*lumbar*) part of the back is the area that is usually referred to when talking about chronic back pain.

Acute back pain is actually the most common type of lower back pain. Acute back pain may come on suddenly and can be very severe, lasting a few minutes or hours, or a few days or weeks. It may be caused by heavy lifting at work or by an injury resulting from an auto accident. In reality, in most cases of acute back pain, the cause cannot be found. Nevertheless, about 80 percent of those with acute back pain can expect to find relief within two weeks.

If you have back pain and also suffer from any of these warning signs, then you should contact your doctor immediately: pain that wakes you up at night, pain that travels down a leg, pain made worse with cough or sneeze, loss of bowl or bladder control, or difficulty in passing urine or having a bowel movement.

If acute back pain continues and lasts for more than three months then it is called *chronic back pain*. This lower back pain can be constant. It can be felt as sharp, dull or burning pain and is often deep or aching. Chronic back pain can travel down either or both legs, especially the back of the legs. Along with the pain can be felt numbness or tingling sensations in the back, hips, and legs.

Unlike the acute form, back pain that becomes chronic is much harder to control in the long term. The pain may cause problems in all areas of a person's life. Sufferers of chronic back pain know the serious limitations and even devastating results it can have. All areas of daily activity can be affected: work, family relationships, personality, sexual function, and general health.

There are many different causes of chronic back pain, but most persons suffer with one of the common forms. The most common cause is thought to be due to pain coming from the muscles, tendons, ligaments, and the joints of the lower spine. The exact reason for the origin of pain in these areas is not known.

Roger N., a forty-two-year-old manager of an appliance store, spoke of struggling off and on with back pain for most of his adult life— over twenty years! He went through three back surgeries to repair a disc problem and even tried a special clinic to end the worsening pain.

"The most difficult problem I have is that I am the main breadwinner for our family. If I have to leave my job, what will we do?" Roger said. "I wake up every day with some pain, and by the end of the day the pain is relentless. The greater the pain, the less my ability to get along with my employees, customers, and family."

Far fewer persons are affected by chronic than by acute back pain. But the smaller numbers affected by chronic back pain incur most of the healthcare expense. Some estimate the total cost at $50 billion to $70 billion when healthcare, wages, and other factors are counted. It is the most common cause of disability in men and women under forty-five. This is discouraging, but the positive side is that if a small improvement could be made in alleviating the suffering of chronic back pain, then a large gain in costs might be possible.

CHRONIC BACK PAIN CAN BE DISCOURAGING

Constant back pain gradually affects the entire person. The pain can make many daily activities, such as standing, walking, sitting, and even coughing, unbearable. This constant pain leads to less activity. Pain can interrupt good sleep patterns, resulting in fatigue even in the morning. This fatigue adds to a low frustration level with easy irritation over minor problems, and it makes it difficult to get along with others, including family.

With the constant pain, it is easy to get discouraged and depressed; depression in turn may create even more problems and increased withdrawal from activities. If pain medicines such as narcotics are used, these may actually make depression worsen, especially if taken too frequently.

THE CYCLE OF PAIN

Another way to look at the problem of chronic pain is to imagine a cycle of pain. The never-ending pain causes less and less activity.

Decreased activity causes more discouragement, which in turn leads to depression. Depression results in further decrease in activities. The more inactive a person becomes, the less he or she will exercise, and the more likely it is that pain will increase. As you will see, many of the ways in which this pain cycle is attacked are directed at these parts of the cycle.

Treatment of this form of chronic pain is very important because the earlier treatment is begun, the better the chances are of improvement. This means that the effort and treatment applied during the early stages of chronic back pain can give better results than the same amount of treatment and effort later. But it is never too late to try to gain some improvement in pain and loss of activity due to chronic back pain. By following the steps given in chapter 3, you can begin today to win with your chronic pain and put an end to the cycle of discomfort and despair.

TRIGGER POINTS

Trigger points are small, localized areas in muscles and tendons (which attach muscles to bones) that are very tender. The pain may also be felt in other areas away from the tender trigger point which may be only slightly tender. The trigger areas occur at predictable locations over the back and hips. There may also be trigger areas in the neck, shoulders, knees, and elbows (see figure 2.1).

The diagnosis of trigger points is made by examination, which assists in finding these extremely tender areas of pain. Areas of tenderness around the back, hips, and shoulders may also produce pain that travels and is felt in other areas of the body (see figure 2.2). For example, a trigger area around the lower back or hip may cause you to feel pain down your leg. This can at times appear much like the pressure on a nerve from a ruptured disc.

X-rays are normal; that is, the condition does not show up on X-rays unless there are other problems present. These trigger areas can happen independently, or they can cause pain along with the discomfort of arthritis, ruptured disc, or any number of other problems from which back pain arises. Treatment of these trigger areas can often significantly improve the pain relief, even when one of the other problems causing back pain is still present.

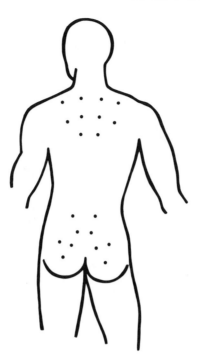

Figure 2.1. Trigger areas are a common source of chronic back pain.

RUPTURED (HERNIATED) DISC

Here there is pressure on a nerve in the back, usually the lower (lumbar) spine. It is most often caused by rupture of a disc with the disc material causing pressure on a nerve as it leaves the spine but before it travels down the leg. There may be severe pain along with numbness and tingling that travels down the leg to the foot. Weakness of the leg or foot may also occur (see figure 2.3).

With a ruptured or herniated disc, the pain may be sharp or dull. It may be felt more on the right or left or even in the center of the back. It may be worse with coughing or sneezing and usually interrupts sleep. If there is pressure on the nerves to the bladder or bowels, there can be some difficulty with incontinence.

If the pain does not improve over a day or weeks then testing by using CT (Computed Tomographic) scan or MRI (Magnetic Resonance Imaging) of the lumbar spine can show the ruptured disc.

A CT scan is a painless test that can show the spine in great detail. It can display ruptured discs, abnormal blood vessels, and other problems.

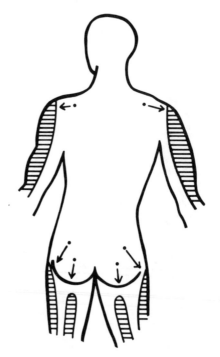

Figure 2.2. The pain from trigger areas can travel to other areas.

It shows ruptured discs in 80 percent or more of the cases. The CT scan involves a modest amount of radiation.

MRI is also a painless test and shows greater detail than a CT scan, allowing for an earlier detection of some spinal abnormalities. This test can show a ruptured disc in over 90 percent of the cases. The MRI test is more expensive than the CT scan but does not involve radiation (see figure 2.4).

Most persons with ruptured disc improve without surgery when the treatment plan is followed. But if medical treatment does not control the pain, tingling and muscle weakness, then surgery could be necessary.

LUMBAR STENOSIS

At times there may be a gradual narrowing of the bones around the spinal canal, which contains the nerve roots after they leave the spinal cord. If the narrowing continues, there may be pressure on these nerves—a condition called *lumbar stenosis.* A common cause of this is *osteoarthritis,* the "wear-and-tear" form of arthritis. This type of arthritis is

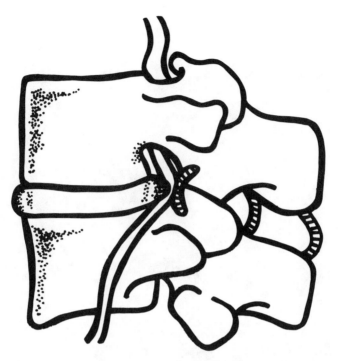

Figure 2.3. A ruptured disc can affect the back and the legs.

caused by wearing of the cartilage that cushions the joints and results in wearing of the joints themselves. There may also be ruptured discs present, causing additional narrowing.

The pain of lumbar stenosis can often be felt in both legs when walking. Usually the pain stops when you stop walking. The distance walked before pain begins may gradually become shorter and shorter. Much like a ruptured disc, lumbar stenosis can be diagnosed by MRI or CT scan of the lumbar spine. Surgery to relieve the pressure on the nerves causing pain is commonly needed to obtain excellent relief, but some patients improve without surgery.

INJURIES

Injuries on the job or as a result of automobile accidents are common causes of back pain, especially the chronic variety. The most common problems found in these cases are pain from the muscles, tendons, and other soft tissues; trigger areas of pain around the lower back; and ruptured discs in the lower spine. Injuries resulting in lower back pain

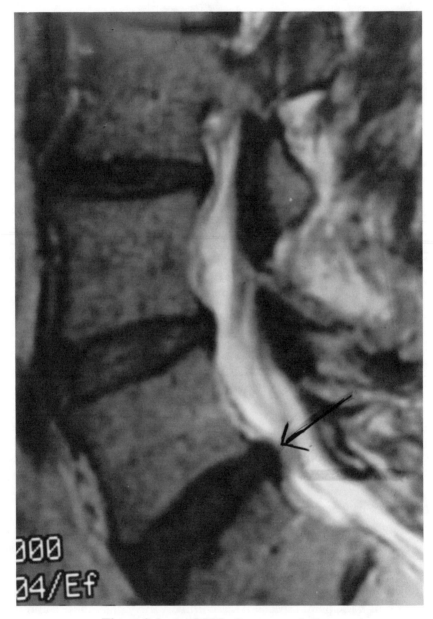

Figure 2.4. An MRI of a ruptured disc

are the major part of the total expense of back pain, which costs from $50 to $75 billion yearly.

Diagnosis of the causes of back pain after injuries can be difficult because there may be several causes contributing to the pain. It may indeed be necessary to seek more than one opinion in complicated cases. But proper diagnosis will allow not only treatment of each individual cause but better pain control.

ARTHRITIS AND CHRONIC BACK PAIN

Arthritis, inflammation in and around the joints causes pain and stiffness that becomes worse when the joints are used. Although we think of arthritis as forming in the hands and limbs, it attacks the back as well as other joints. People with arthritis frequently complain of stiffness on rising in the morning. Lethargy and fatigue may be severe with many forms of arthritis and may even equal the pain in the limitations they impose on sufferers. There can even be fever, weight loss, and other problems along with the pain and stiffness.

Many types of arthritis can cause chronic back pain. There are over one hundred types of arthritis, the most common type being osteoarthritis. Pain from osteoarthritis in the back is usually worse with standing or walking. The pain does not usually travel down the legs. A few minutes of stiffness in the back may be noticed when waking in the morning before "loosening up" for the day. The sufferer may also feel stiff after sitting in one position for more than a few minutes.

The diagnosis of osteoarthritis can be made after discussion and examination with X-rays which usually show narrowing of the joints (see figure 2.5).

OSTEOPOROSIS AND CHRONIC BACK PAIN

Osteoporosis means thinning of the bones. After age thirty or so, the bones become gradually thinner, although there is no outward way to tell if this is happening. If the bones become thin enough, they may break (fracture) more easily, even following mild injuries. This is most common in women but it can occur in men, especially those over the age of fifty. There are actually known risk factors that can predict if you have a greater chance of osteoporosis and fractures (see figure 2.6). Up to 80 percent of women over age sixty-five have osteoporosis, but

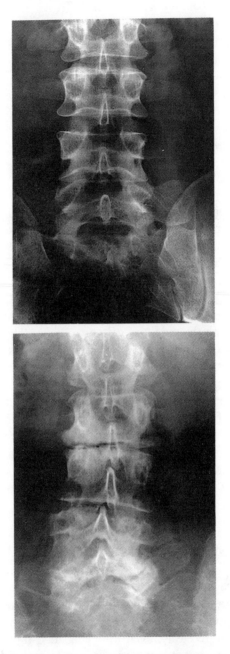

Figure 2.5. X-rays of the spine can show the changes from osteoarthritis. The X-ray on the top is normal. The X-ray on the bottom shows arthritis of the spine.

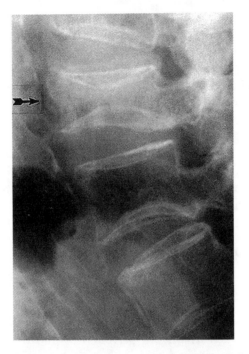

Figure 2.6. X-ray of a compression fracture of the spine

most do not know it until they have a fracture! Now a simple test is available to detect osteoporosis before it causes fractures.

A common area of fracture is in the spine, especially the lower back. The fracture is called a *compression fracture* and may cause severe pain (see figure 2.6). As the bones become thinner, more bones in the spine may have fractures, causing even more pain. This can happen after minor lifting or even as a result of the weight of the body when standing with no injury at all. Twenty-five percent or more of women over age sixty-five develop fractures in the spine.

The thinner the bones become, the more likely fractures are to occur. With each compression fracture, the spine becomes a little shorter. For this reason, osteoporosis is the most common cause of loss of height as we grow older. It is also the most common cause of hip fracture in older persons.

One seventy-year-old woman told of bending down to tie her grandson's shoe when she suddenly felt unbearable pain in her back. After some tests were run, the woman was found to have a fracture due to osteoporosis. She started a treatment program immediately for the osteoporosis, and now is able to be active once more.

A retired man described how he had severe back pain after moving furniture in his den. X-rays showed a fracture in the spine. He is now in treatment and working to prevent further bone loss and fractures.

With newer treatments available, we need no longer simply watch these fractures happen. There are easy steps that can be taken to increase the strength of the bones and to try to prevent future fractures. These steps are discussed on pp. 82–83.

Hip fractures from osteoporosis are dangerous because they can cause disability and significantly reduce a person's independence. Up to 20 percent of older patients who have hip fractures may die within the following year, half do not walk as well again, and many require nursing home care.

RISK FACTORS FOR OSTEOPOROSIS

1. Lack of a Regular Exercise Program

It has been known for years that bones become weaker when activity is very limited, such as when a person is confined to bed for a long period of time. Activity and exercise, especially weight-bearing exercise, stimulates bones to become stronger. Without such activity, bones become less dense and weaker.

Lack of regular exercise, especially weight-bearing exercise, greatly increases the chances of osteoporosis. But this can be easily managed with a simple walking program. Most of the patients we see with fractures due to osteoporosis were not aware that walking could improve bone strength.

Exercises to build other muscles that give support to the body are also important. Stronger muscles give more support to the bones. In fact, it has been shown in some cases that the stronger the back muscles, the stronger the bones of the back. Just follow the guide for exercises as shown in chapter 4.

2. Menopause in Women, Especially Early Menopause

The risk of osteoporosis is much higher in women after the age of menopause, which occurs naturally between the ages of forty-five and fifty-five, or even earlier if the ovaries are removed by surgery.

Ovaries are the female organs that produce one of the female hormones, estrogen. The female hormone system, including estrogen, is important in bone formation. The level of estrogen drops at menopause, which is a major contributor to thinning of the bones and osteoporosis. This risk factor can be detected early and treated with the steps discussed on pp. 82–83.

3. Being Forty Years of Age or Older

There is a gradual decrease in the total amount of bone formed by our bodies compared to the amount of bone removed after we reach maturity. This commonly leads to a gradual thinning of bones. This bone loss may continue as we get older. By age sixty-five, up to 80 percent of women may have osteoporosis!

4. Being Female

The gradual loss of bone that occurs as we grow older happens more rapidly in women than in men. This is due mainly to the loss of the hormone estrogen in women at menopause. Being aware of this fact can help alert you to the need for prevention and early detection of osteoporosis.

5. Being White

Osteoporosis is more common in people of the Caucasian race. African-Americans have denser bones and a less rapid loss of bone once this process begins. White women have about twice as many fractures of the hip due to osteoporosis as African-American women. Indeed, the rate of bone loss and risk of osteoporosis is highest in white women and lowest in African-American men.

6. Cigarette Smoking

The risk of osteoporosis is twice as high in smokers. Osteoporosis occurs earlier and continues to increase more rapidly in those who smoke cigarettes. On the positive side, once you are aware of this increased risk, you may decrease that risk by one-half simply by stopping smoking.

7. Other Family Members with Osteoporosis

There is a higher risk of osteoporosis if you have biological family members who are affected. The reasons are not known, but it is probably due to the inherited genetic program which increases the risk. If you have a family member who has had fractures from osteoporosis, *you may also be at higher risk.*

8. Being Underweight for Your Height

Women who are underweight often develop osteoporosis earlier than others. Those who are overweight actually have less risk. The reasons for this are not completely understood.

9. Heavy Alcohol Use

Drinking alcohol in heavy amounts causes a higher risk of osteoporosis. The exact amount of alcohol needed to cause this higher risk is not known; however, moderate amounts such as one to two ounces of 80 proof distilled liquor, one to two 12 oz. cans of beer, or a half bottle of wine a day do not increase the risk. As with smoking, reducing alcohol consumption can lessen the risk of osteoporosis.

10. Medications

Some medications taken for other medical problems may actually increase your chance of osteoporosis. The most common of these are the cortisone-like drugs. In higher doses or over a period of years, these can increase the risk of bone thinning. A low dose or taking the drug for a brief time usually would not increase the risk.

These medicines may be needed for other serious problems such as lung diseases, asthma, and other diseases. Using the lowest possible dose for the shortest amount of time can help to minimize the effect of these medications.

11. Certain Medical Problems

Lung diseases such as emphysema and chronic bronchitis can increase the risk of osteoporosis. By knowing this fact, you can take steps to help prevent osteoporosis or to detect it as early as possible to allow treatment.

Rheumatoid arthritis causes pain and swelling in the joints, including the hands, wrists, elbows, shoulders, knees, ankles, and feet. This arthritis can be severe and crippling and also increases the risk of osteoporosis and fractures. Fractures can make the arthritis situation even worse and interfere with treatment plans. Knowing that rheumatoid arthritis can increase the chance of osteoporosis can allow you to take steps for prevention and treatment at the earliest stages when it can be most effective.

12. Low Calcium in the Diet

A diet low in calcium (contained in dairy and other food products or taken easily as a supplement) also increases over time the chance of osteoporosis by allowing less bone formation. With loss of bone formation osteoporosis occurs more quickly.

Adults should take 1000 mg calcium daily between diet and supplement. Women after menopause should increase their calcium intake to 1500 mg each day. When weight is a concern, a supplement is an easy way to be sure of enough calcium without the worry of extra calories in dairy products.

MORE THAN ONE CAUSE

It is very common to see persons with more than one contributing cause of back pain. This makes it harder to control the pain, but not at all impossible. A very common combination of problems is from an injury on the job and trigger areas of pain in the back, at times combined with osteoarthritis in the lower spine. If these different causes are recognized and treated separately, the chances of improvement and pain control increase greatly.

Another very common combination of causes of chronic back pain is pain due to osteoarthritis in the spine, trigger areas of pain in the soft tissues, and osteoporosis with a compression fracture in the spine. Each of these causes can be identified. Different treatment is available for each. Effective treatment of each cause can greatly improve control of pain and allow greater movement.

OSTEOARTHRITIS

Osteoarthritis has been called the "wear and tear" arthritis. The cartilage becomes worn and less efficient in cushioning the joints. There can be pain, stiffness, swelling, and warmth in the joints that become harder to use. Osteoarthritis is most common after age fifty but can occur earlier in life.

Osteoarthritis can affect joints that bear weight over the years, such as the knees, hips, or lower back as well as other joints. Because of this, it is a common cause of pain in these areas. Osteoarthritis is also a common cause of chronic knee, hip, or back pain. The pain is usually worse with activity such as standing or walking, but may eventually be present all the time.

Injuries to joints can also cause osteoarthritis. For example, a football player may have pain and stiffness in a knee from osteoarthritis years after an injury. The problem occurs as the cartilage becomes damaged and worn away. This results in pain, swelling, and stiffness in the joint.

Juanita, a fifty-five-year-old high school teacher, was faced with early retirement due to the chronic pain of osteoarthritis. She told of feeling only slight pain on rising in the morning; but after teaching five English classes a day, the pain was almost unbearable at night.

"I could hardly get through my last class because the pain was so intense," Juanita said. "Some days I would give the students a reading assignment so I could sit down and take the pressure off my hip and knees."

After starting a treatment program as outlined in chapter 3, including medication, moist heat, exercise, and losing fifteen pounds, Juanita was able to postpone her retirement and now looks forward to teaching for many more years. A year ago, she could barely walk into the class-room. Now Juanita is able to stand all day, without pain, and still have the energy to enjoy her evenings with the family. She tells of joining a bowling league and not hurting for the first time in ten years!

Early diagnosis of osteoarthritis is extremely important, since there are good treatments available. These begin with a basic medical treatment program as shown in chapter 3. If there is not enough improvement, then other treatments, including surgery, may give excellent pain relief. It may not be necessary to suffer with the pain of osteoarthritis after proper diagnosis and treatment.

OTHER TYPES OF ARTHRITIS

After osteoarthritis, the next most common group of arthritis conditions are those that cause inflammation of the linings of the joints. The joints usually become painful, swollen, and warm and may be red and tender to the touch. There are many different types of inflammatory arthritis, but the most common is rheumatoid arthritis.

Rheumatoid Arthritis

Rheumatoid arthritis, whose cause is not known, affects over ten million Americans. It strikes women more often than men and can begin at almost any age. People with rheumatoid arthritis experience pain, swelling and stiffness in the hands, wrists, elbows, shoulders, knees, ankles, feet, or other joints in various combinations. Morning stiffness may be severe and last for hours, often with severe lethargy and fatigue that prevents activity. Fever, weight loss, and other problems may arise.

Rheumatoid arthritis can cause destruction of the bones near joints, as well as deformities and crippling. Along with the arthritis, there is often chronic pain in the joints. The pain may make it difficult to work, dress, walk, or even use a knife and fork.

Since there is good treatment available for rheumatoid arthritis, it is important to have the diagnosis made as early as possible. There is a better result with earlier treatment, especially with the new medications available. It is now hoped that early diagnosis combined with effective medications and other treatments may delay or prevent crippling and deformity. Also, the more the arthritis can be controlled, the less severe the physical limitation will be.

Ankylosing Spondylitis

This type of arthritis affects men more than women and often begins in the teenage years and on into young adulthood. It begins gradually with pain in the lower back. What may seem like a strain or injury continues; there is usually stiffness on rising in the morning, and the pain worsens with prolonged inactivity.* It is common for young men to have this cause of back pain for years, thinking it is an injury or other problem.

Over a few years the pain may gradually be felt in the middle, then the upper part of the back. Eventually there can be pain in the neck. The spine may become stiffer so that movement is limited, especially in the lower back. This can restrict some activities, especially bending. About one-half of all persons affected with ankylosing spondylitis contract arthritis in the shoulders, hips, or other joints.

Other problems can go along with this form of arthritis, including eye inflammation (*iritis*), which can affect vision if not treated. Ninety percent of those with ankylosing spondylitis have a positive blood test

---

*Usually, in a back injury, the pain is *less* severe with inactivity.

for a marker called HLA-B27 antigen. This marker is inherited and increases the chances of developing ankylosing spondylitis. It is thought that those who inherit this marker may develop arthritis after contact with something in their environment that triggers the arthritis. This could be an infection or other unknown contact.

It is important to diagnose this type of arthritis because proper treatment may help improve the pain and stiffness and allow a much greater range of activity. It is also very important to maintain exercises and other steps to help prevent loss of mobility and a stiffness of the spine and a stooped posture. Early diagnosis and treatment offer an excellent chance for prevention of disability. See your doctor if you have persistent lower back pain.

Fibromyalgia and "Soft Tissue Pain"

These problems cause pain and stiffness in the back, neck, shoulders, arms, and legs. There is often a feeling of stiffness all over. The pain in fibromyalgia is also very widespread over the body. Sleep is disturbed and often interrupted. There is frequent morning stiffness, fatigue, depression, and headache. In fibromyalgia the pain is felt all over, but there are more localized areas of soft tissue pain. This condition can affect the shoulders, hips, back, legs, and arms.

In fibromyalgia, there is usually no joint swelling, but the pain may be very prominent. Activities can usually be performed, but with pain. There are many areas over the neck, back, arms, and legs called trigger areas; these are very tender to the touch. Pressure on one of these tender areas may "trigger" pain felt in other areas. Fibromyalgia may also occur along with one of the other one hundred types of arthritis (see figure 2.7).

The diagnosis of fibromyalgia is important if sufferers are to understand the pain and secure treatment. Unfortunately, proper diagnosis can be difficult because there are no specific tests available, and X-rays do not usually show signs of the condition. It may require several examinations to make sure that no other problems have been overlooked.

Since fibromyalgia originates in the muscles, tendons, and ligaments rather than the joints or bones, it can cause considerable discomfort even though there may be no joint pain or swelling and no other signs of inflammation. With the right approach, treatment is possible (see chapter 3).

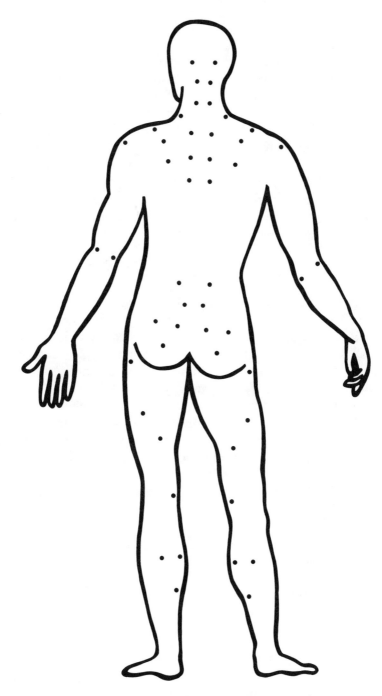

Figure 2.7. Trigger areas of fibromyalgia

Bursitis

Inflammation from one of the bursa sacs that allow muscles to move smoothly results in bursitis. Bursitis causes pain upon movement of a muscle or tendon around a joint such as the shoulder, hip, or knee. This pain can make it very difficult to move the shoulder or hip. Also, it can cause severe pain when lying down on the side of the affected area, which can interfere with sleep.

Bursitis most commonly attacks areas around the shoulders, hips, and knees but many other areas, including the buttocks, may be involved. When pain becomes chronic, it can render the joint stiff and efforts to move the joint may become permanently limited. Treatment is available once the diagnosis is made (see chapter 3).

Tendinitis

Tendinitis is caused by inflammation of a tendon, which attaches muscle to bone. This condition can cause pain while people are at rest but usually it is more severe when the muscle is used. "Tennis elbow" and "golfers' elbow" are common forms of tendinitis, which can develop separately, on its own, or along with other types of arthritis.

Bursitis and tendinitis are commonly found along with other causes of chronic pain. Since these also are treatable, it is helpful to be sure that each area is given proper treatment (as shown in chapter 3). Even though treatment of these portions of a person's complete pain picture gives us much to hope for, it may not eliminate the entire pain problem. We often find that removing a part of the pain that is treatable can help make the total pain more tolerable. If this also allows more exercise and activity, then it may have an even greater total effect on chronic pain.

There are many other less common types of arthritis that cause chronic pain. Most types of arthritis are treatable, so people should not let arthritis keep them from winning with chronic pain. If a doctor's opinion is required, a rheumatologist (an arthritis specialist) may need to be consulted.

CHRONIC HEADACHES

Some surveys have reported that 70 to 90 percent of all women and men have headaches. Of this number, 40 to 50 percent of women and men report headaches that they regard as disabling. Most common headaches are brief and mild, but others are frequent and severe. Headaches can be horrible whether or not the underlying cause is serious or life-threatening. And when the pain is severe, it can be disabling no matter what the cause.

If a headache is severe or persistent, medical advice should be sought, since this can be the first sign of a more serious problem. Fortunately, most headaches are not of a life-threatening nature, although the pain itself can be very limiting.

MUSCLE CONTRACTION HEADACHES

Muscle contraction headaches are also called tension headaches, with tightening of the muscles of the neck and head that cause the pain. This is common in times of stress or when the person is tired. These headaches may be mild and easily relieved by rest or by taking an over-the-counter pain medication such as Advil.® If these headaches happen daily or several times a day, they can significantly limit daily activities (see figure 2.8).

This type of headache may feel like a dull pain accompanied by tightness, a band of pressure in or around the head. The pain may extend over the top of the head to the front. The neck or jaws may also feel pain if there is tightness of the muscles in these areas, too. This variety of headache afflicts both women and men, and it is common for family members to have similar headaches.

When this type of headache becomes very frequent or constant, there may also be a great deal of stress present along with depression or other problems. The sufferer may experience sleep deprivation, eating problems, and fatigue. Since stress can be managed and depression treated, it is important that the problems that may be causing the headache be properly diagnosed. Once these problems are isolated, the headaches may also be treated more effectively.

HEADACHES FROM ARTHRITIS

Arthritis in the neck can be a cause of headache. The most common type of arthritis in this case would be osteoarthritis (the "wear and tear" arthritis), but rheumatoid arthritis and ankylosing spondylitis can also cause headaches. For those who experience these headaches there is commonly pain and tenderness in the muscles of the neck that can

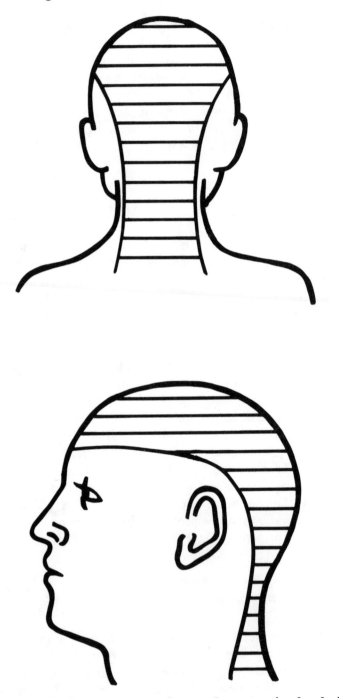

Figure 2.8. Common areas of a muscle contraction headache

contribute to the pain. Treatment for each of these individual conditions is available once the cause is discovered.

VASCULAR HEADACHES

Vascular headaches are usually caused by enlargement (dilation) of arteries in and around the head, which causes the pain. The most common type is migraine headache. Migraines affect an estimated 10 to 20 million people or as many as 16 percent of women and 9 percent of men. These may last a few hours or a few days, and can be dull, throbbing, constant, and severe. They may happen only occasionally or may repeat within days. Migraines are most often (but not always) on one side of the head and usually felt in the front or side of the head.

Other problems beside simple headache can accompany migraines. Nausea or vomiting usually occur, and occasionally the sufferer will have diarrhea. Lights and a bright room may make the headache much worse. In some forms of migraine headache (called the classic migraine), the person may experience blind spots, see light flashes in their vision, or notice other visual changes before the onset of the headache.

Other types of vascular headaches include those caused by high blood pressure (hypertension), fever, some chemicals, alcohol use, and some foods. For example, some persons are sensitive to certain wines, cheese, monosodium glutamate in Chinese food, or nitrites in hot dogs. Since each of these vascular type headaches may have available treatment, it is important first to identify the problem. Seek the advice of your physician.

OTHER CAUSES OF HEADACHE

Problems inside the head can cause headaches. A common concern in patients with headaches is whether there may be a *brain tumor.* Headaches may be the first sign in less than one-third of diagnosed brain tumors. There are usually other signs of a brain tumor that can be found on examination by your doctor. If this worries you, let your doctor know so that this concern can be eliminated quickly.

Headaches can accompany pain in the jaw from TMJ syndrome (discussed on pp. 52–53), injuries to the head, sinus infection, and inflammation of the nerves and arteries. Diseases of the eye, ear, nose, or teeth are possible but less common causes of chronic headaches. Patients are sometimes concerned that their headaches are the sign of a stroke, but this is a very uncommon cause of chronic headaches.

DIAGNOSING THE CAUSES OF HEADACHES

In addition to a general discussion and physical examination, your doctor may ask you to have a few other tests to help find the cause of the pain. In most cases only a few tests are needed to provide the answer. Blood tests in addition to one or more of the following procedures may be needed.

X-Rays

In some cases, X-rays of the neck or skull may be taken. In cases of arthritis or injury to the head or neck, these have proved helpful in finding the problem. Some other medical problems may become apparent as well.

Computed Tomographic (CT) Scan and
Magnetic Resonance Imaging (MRI)

Computed tomographic (CT) scan of the head is a painless test usually done in the X-ray department of a clinic or hospital. It allows greater detail of the brain than an X-ray. It is painless and involves a modest amount of radiation.

A CT scan can isolate tumors, abnormal blood vessels, infections, and other problems. Usually if the headache is severe, or if there is suspicion of a brain tumor, then a CT scan will be requested.

Magnetic Resonance Imaging (MRI) is a test also done in the X-ray deparment of a hospital or clinic. It is painless and does not involve radiation as the CT scan does. It is more expensive than a CT scan.

MRI may be able to show some areas of the brain more clearly than a CT scan. Talk to your doctor so that proper diagnosis of your headaches can be achieved and treatment started.

TMJ (TEMPOROMANDIBULAR JOINT) SYNDROME

The most common source of pain in the jaw and nearby areas in the face and neck has been called the Temporomandibular Joint (TMJ) Syndrome. Pain can be felt in the jaw just in front of the ear, or it may be felt over the side of the face and head, then extend to the neck. The pain is often constant and worse with chewing, and there may be a sensation of cracking in the jaw when the mouth is opened. Pain may limit the opening of the jaw. The jaw may move to one side when it is opened. Headaches are common along with the jaw pain (see figure 2.9).

Jaw pain and the TMJ Syndrome are common problems. Surveys show that 12 to 20 percent of people are affected in some populations. This problem is common in younger adults but actually happens less often after age fifty.

The pain may be due to arthritis in the jaw joint itself (the temporomandibular joint) from one of the many different types of arthritis, including osteoarthritis and rheumatoid arthritis. If there has been an injury to the jaw, such as from a fall or broken jaw, the cartilage of the joint may be damaged, which can result in osteoarthritis of the TMJ.

Dental problems and bite abnormalities can cause TMJ pain as well. If there is any imbalance in the way teeth come together, there may be higher pressure in one or both jaws and temporomandibular joints. If there are teeth missing on one side, there will be an abnormal chewing motion with higher pressure on one side. This can cause more stress on one side of the jaw. The unbalanced pressures and stress on the TMJ then cause more pain.

Ear diseases can cause pain that feels more like jaw pain than ear pain, even though the problem is in the ear. Sometimes the pain in the ear is such that cotton tips or other objects are used to try to clean the ear. Specific treatment of the ear disease is needed in this case to help the jaw pain. Don't put objects in your ear if you have ear pain. See your doctor.

Stress Affects Jaw Pain

Stress can also cause pain in the jaw area. This can result in more tension in the muscles of the jaw, the face, and the neck, which causes more spasms and still more pain. Clenching the teeth during the day or grinding the teeth at night can result from stress, thereby increasing the tension on muscles around the jaw. This is a common cause of TMJ pain.*

---

*See chapter 7 for ways to reduce your stress, and practice the relaxation response given in chapter 5.

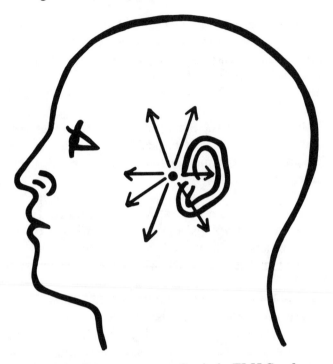

Figure 2.9. Common areas of pain in TMJ Syndrome

It is also common to find pain in other areas along with the TMJ. The pain may be felt in the neck or head and may extend to the shoulders and upper back. In these cases the TMJ pain may be one part of a wider area of pain in the muscles, tendons, and ligaments (the "soft tissues"). This may be part of the larger chronic pain problem of fibromyalgia.

With the "soft tissue" pain and fibromyalgia, there may be trigger areas around the jaws, face, and neck (see figure 2.10). These are localized areas of tenderness in muscles, tendons, and other "soft tissues," which may trigger pain felt in other areas of the face and neck. A very common complaint in these persons is headache.

Many people who suffer from this form of chronic pain show signs of stress and may show signs of depression. Treatment of the trigger areas along with any other medical problems and depression can give much better pain relief.

Inflammation of the nerves that supply the face, infections of the face, and tumors are less common causes of pain in the jaw and face. Though these causes of pain are not as common, they are still important to note because they may be treated specifically. Sinus infections, dental and gum infections, and abscesses can also cause pain in the jaw and face. These can usually be treated with antibiotics.

Diagnosis of chronic jaw and facial pain can be very difficult. Doctors will first make sure no other underlying diseases are present. If more than one problem is found to be causing the pain, it may take the effort of several experienced doctors to solve the problem. The best answers in cases of severe chronic jaw and facial pain may be found by including dental evaluation along with other testing. Then treatment for each separate cause of pain can be planned for the most complete relief.

CHRONIC NECK PAIN

Pain in the neck is so common that one out of ten Americans suffers from it at any given time. Over half of all persons questioned remember having an attack of stiff or painful neck. Most of the time the neck pain is acute and goes away within a few days or weeks. Those persons who continue to have neck pain can find this to be a major disruption of their lives. Daily movements—dressing, driving, eating, working—may all become very painful and limited when neck pain attacks.

If you find that neck pain is severe or lasts more than a few days with no apparent cause, then see your doctor. A few of the most common causes of chronic neck pain are listed below.

NECK SPRAIN

Pain can happen after a sprain of the muscles, tendons, or ligaments of the neck. This can come from an injury in sports, an automobile accident, or may even happen as a result of poor posture or overuse of the neck at work. When there is a known specific injury, the neck pain and stiffness usually happens within days of the event.

The pain may be mild at first, but may gradually worsen over days or weeks. It is best to treat the neck sprain early to increase the chances of better pain control. The longer the sprain lasts, the more attention it should be given to be sure proper treatment is continued.

The more severe the injury, the more likely it is that there may be damage to the muscles, tendons, and ligaments in the neck. A good example of this is the "whiplash" injury to the neck in an automobile accident. The head is suddenly thrown backwards or forwards, which is followed by a sudden rebound movement in the opposite direction.

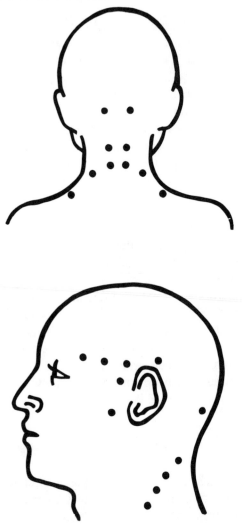

Figure 2.10. Trigger areas in the jaws, face, and neck

The stronger the force on the neck, the more injury to the "soft tissues" and more severe the pain may be. Other areas in the neck and head can sustain injury, including injury to the jaw (temporomandibular) joint or other structures. This could include dislocations of joints or small fractures in the bones of the spine. In severe injuries there may be damage to the nerves in the neck or in the spinal cord. These are the kinds of injuries that can lead to chronic neck pain. It is vital that proper diagnosis and treatment commence as early as possible.

Trigger points are a common cause of chronic neck pain. These localized areas around muscles and other areas in the neck become painful when pressure is applied. The pain can travel and may produce painful senstions in other areas as well. Such dispersal of pain can occur after an injury, or with arthritis in the neck, with overwork of the muscles, or with stress.

Trigger areas may cause pain that travels down one arm and can mimic pressure on a nerve in the neck. Treatment is available for this problem (see chapter 3). If left untreated, these trigger areas may be very long-lasting and a major cause of chronic neck pain.

ARTHRITIS IN THE NECK

Many forms of arthritis that cause pain and stiffness in joints can affect the neck. The most common type is osteoarthritis (the "wear and tear" arthritis). The cartilage of the joints between the bones in the neck becomes worn or less efficient, which can result in pain and stiffness when moving the neck. It is most common in persons over age fifty or after injuries to the neck. There is often a feeling of stiffness on rising in the morning, though it lasts only a few minutes. There may be pain and stiffness from osteoarthritis in joints other than the neck, such as the knees, hips, or hands.

This type of arthritis can usually be diagnosed after discussion, examination, and X-rays of the neck. There is good treatment available in most cases, so this common problem should not be overlooked as a cause of chronic neck pain.

Two other types of arthritis may commonly cause chronic neck pain. *Rheumatoid arthritis* causes pain, swelling, and stiffness in the hands, wrists, feet, and other joints. It can also attack the neck, where it causes pain, stiffness, headaches, and makes movement of the neck very painful. In most cases the person is already aware that there is arthritis in other joints. Treatment is available to control the arthritis and can usually give relief from neck pain. In severe cases, however, the spine may become so damaged that surgery is needed.

Ankylosing spondylitis, a form of arthritis we discussed earlier, especially attacks the spine, beginning in the lower back and gradually moving to the upper back and neck. There is usually pain and stiffness in the spine before the neck is affected. The neck may be very stiff and difficult to move when driving or while engaged in other activities needed during the day. Many persons who suffer from this type of arthritis must deal with serious chronic neck pain. The condition is usually diagnosed by X-rays of the neck. There is no cure, but treatment to control the pain and retain use of the neck is available.

Other causes such as cancerous tumors can affect the neck although, as causes of chronic neck pain, these are not common. These problems can usually be discovered through X-rays, bone scan, and MRI of the cervical spine. If you worry that cancer is the root cause of your pain, talk with your doctor; tests can be run that will help to eliminate this serious problem as the source of your pain.

NECK PAIN WITH PRESSURE ON A NERVE

This problem is not as common as pressure on a nerve in the lower back, which can cause back and leg pain. There is usually pain in the neck which travels down one or both arms, often to the fingers. There may also be a feeling of numbness or tingling that may also travel down the arm. The feeling may be like pins and needles in the arms or feel as if the arm has "fallen asleep." The pain can cause its sufferers to awaken at night and may become worse when the person coughs or sneezes.

The most common cause of pressure on a nerve as it leaves the spinal cord is a ruptured disc in the neck due to osteoarthritis or injury. This ruptured disc can cause severe, even disabling, neck pain. MRI tests of the neck area are a good way to discover pressure on a nerve. Once other more serious problems are eliminated, medical treatment is available and usually successful. Most people do not need surgery to remove pressure on the nerve, but this is an effective treatment when necessary. Your doctor can advise you.

CANCER PAIN

In addition to all of the other problems and suffering that cancer brings with it, pain often interferes with activity and sleep. In fact, the quality of life may be greatly enhanced when the pain of cancer is controlled— with an increase in the person's range of activities, the comfort and enjoyment for both patients and families can greatly improve. This is separate from other problems of treating the underlying cancer itself.

Most important is the correct diagnosis and overall treatment plan for the cancer. This should be directed by your physician, internal medicine specialist, or oncologist (the specialist who deals with cancer and its treatment).

When there is new or changing pain in cancer patients, it is important that the evaluation allow accurate diagnosis of the cause of pain. It is not unusual for a new cause of such pain to be found, which can allow more effective treatment in many cases. The new causes most commonly found include the spread of the cancer to the bone and new problems from nerve pain.

The chronic pain of cancer is mainly due to the direct effects of the cancer on bones and nerves, or to the adverse effects of the cancer treatment. Cancer can invade bones directly, a source of severe pain. Or the cancer can damage nerves in which case the result may be constant pain. There can also be pain after surgery to remove the cancer.

Proper diagnosis of the specific causes of the pain in cancer patient is important. Most causes of pain can be controlled once they are identified.

NERVE PAIN

Pain as the result of damage to nerves is a common cause of chronic pain. Up to one-fourth of all patients seen at one large pain clinic were there for nerve pain. Damage to a nerve can happen in many ways. For example, an injured foot, leg, or hand can physically damage a nerve and lead to chronic pain. Or an infection can cause damage to a nerve. Some diseases such as diabetes mellitus damage nerve endings in ways that are not completely understood but nonetheless cause constant pain.

Rodney L., a sixty-three-year-old minister, told of his feet feeling as if he were walking on "a bed of pins and needles" all day. He was found to have neuropathy, or nerve damage, which is a serious complication of diabetes. One form of nerve pain can even cause pain to be felt in a leg after that leg has been amputated!

If you suffer from nerve pain, there are some facts that are helpful to know. Of the many causes of nerve pain, most result in very similar types of pain. In other words, two very different causes of nerve damage often cause painful sensations that seem just alike.

Pain caused by nerve damage is often burning, shooting, or stabbing. A painful foot or leg may actually be *less* sensitive to the touch most of the time even though it is the source of much more pain. Or else, lightly touching the painful area may cause pain while holding the area more firmly may help relieve the discomfort. Many people find that their nerve pain is worse when they are angry or under stress but that it improves when they are more relaxed. The skin in a painful area may feel warmer or cooler than other areas of the body.

A few of the most common causes of nerve pain are the following:

Infection

Viruses and other infections can bring about nerve pain. Shingles, or herpes zoster, is a typical example of a viral infection of the nerves. Shingles is an infection of nerves by the same virus that causes chicken pox. The virus stays in the body and becomes "reactivated" later in life to cause a rash with pain and blisters. About one-half of cases attack one side of the chest and back. One-fourth attack the face but it can appear anywhere from the face to the foot. It follows the same path as the nerve it infects (see figure 2.11).

The rash may gradually go away over a few weeks, but the pain may last for weeks or even months after the rash has disappeared. About half of those over age sixty develop pain after a bout with shingles. The pain is felt as burning, shooting, or aching, and the skin is usually very tender to touch.

Carpal Tunnel Syndrome

This is an increasingly occurring problem that causes pain, tingling, and numbness in the hand. It is mainly felt in the palm, thumb, and index and middle finger (see figure 2.12). The pain or numbness may be most noticeable at night or when driving a car. Relief may come from moving the hand and wrist for a few minutes. Weakness may occur in the muscles of the hand when the problem has been present there for months or years.

Carpal tunnel syndrome is caused by pressure on the median nerve as it passes through the wrist. There are many different problems that cause pressure on that nerve, but this syndrome often occurs when there has been repetitive use of the wrist and hand, such as typing or other repeated activity. It also can happen when arthritis attacks the wrist.

Carpal tunnel syndrome can last for years. If a basic underlying problem for the condition can be found, then it should be treated. If the pain, numbness, or tingling start to limit your activity or if the muscles of the hand are affected, then treatment is needed to relieve pressure on the nerve.

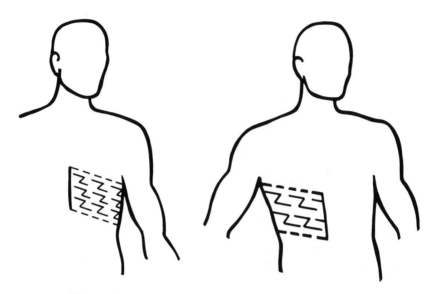

Figure 2.11. An area commonly affected by shingles

Nerve Pain from Diabetes Mellitus

In this condition, damaged nerves in the lower legs and feet create false sensations instead of normal feelings. This results in burning, tingling pain. There may even be a sensation of numbness at times. It happens most commonly in the area of the feet and lower legs which would be covered by a sock or stocking (see figure 2.13). The pain interferes with daily activities such as walking and working. There is often pain at night, which causes the sufferer to awaken from sleep with burning of the soles of the feet. There may be weakness of some of the muscles of the lower legs, which, however, does not cause pain.

Up to 25 percent of diabetics suffer from nerve pain. Half of those who have had diabetes for more than twenty-five years are affected by this neuropathy. It happens more commonly if the blood glucose (sugar) level is not very well controlled. The pain can be very limiting, but treatment is available.

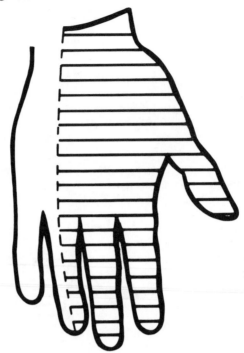

**Figure 2.12. Carpal tunnel syndrome affects
the fingers, thumb, and palm.**

Other Causes

Alcohol

Excessive alcohol use over a long period of time can also cause nerve
pain, usually in the feet and lower legs, similar to that of diabetes mellitus.
This is a result of damage to the nerves in the legs by the alcohol
or by poor nutrition which may be associated with heavy alcohol intake.

Trigeminal Neuralgia

This is severe pain in the face, which feels like stabbing, shooting, or
a shock. It is often triggered by touching a "trigger area" on the face.
This is a less common cause of nerve pain but can be severely limiting.

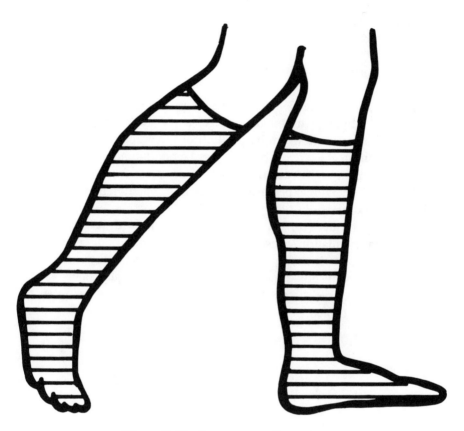

Figure 2.13. Leg neuropathy pattern

Injury

Direct injury (e.g., broken jaw, severe bruising, fractures) to a nerve can cause chronic pain since it damages the nerve's fibers that carry pain and other sensations. Even when the nerve is cut completely it can continue to be a source of pain.

Stroke

After a stroke some of those affected may suffer pain in part or all of an arm, leg, or face. The pain can begin at the time of the stroke in the affected limb or may begin months afterward.

Phantom Limb Pain

This refers to pain that is felt in the location of a limb that has been amputated. Although it sounds strange, it has been found that most amputees have sensations in the position of the amputated limb. Some even feel pain in this area. The pain can be continuous or it can come and go. The pain can be described as mild or severe, burning, stabbing, or shooting. The pains experienced following amputation may fade away after a few months or last for years.

Still other causes of nerve pain include certain drugs, chemicals, poor arterial circulation, cancer, and other less common diseases. Since many of these causes need proper diagnosis and treatment if pain relief is to be found, you should seek out the advice of your physician.

In chapter 3 we discuss how each of these causes of pain can be treated and controlled.

3

A Treatment Plan for Chronic Pain

Once a proper evaluation of the causes of your chronic pain has been conducted, you can start a plan to regain control of your life. It is very important that no shortcuts are made in finding the cause(s) of the pain. If any causes have specific treatment, pain relief and correction of the underlying problem can be accomplished simultaneously. Otherwise, treatment could be started without solving the original problem, giving less chance of ending the chronic pain.

For example, chronic back pain can come from problems with the internal organs. If the pain is caused by kidney or stomach disease, or some other internal organ abnormality, you would want to correct the basic problem, which would then remove the back pain. Rather than begin a program simply to control the chronic back pain, it is necessary first to treat the underlying cause, if at all possible.

Joan T., a fifty-year-old woman, had chronic back pain for four months. She had been evaluated for a ruptured lumbar disc but the tests were negative. Further testing showed that she actually had gall bladder disease, but the back pain was bothering her more than the abdominal pain. After surgery for the gall bladder disease, her chronic back pain went away completely.

Another man came to our clinic with back pain that lasted for six months and that seemed gradually to become worse. When it began keeping him awake for several nights in a row, he sought further help. He was found to have cancer of the prostate gland that had spread to the bones of the spine. After appropriate treatment, he is now free of pain.

PLAN TODAY TO CONTROL YOUR PAIN

Treatment of chronic pain is both easy and difficult. While it may be easy to learn what you need to do, it can be difficult to make yourself stay with the program long enough to see improvement. Make a plan *today* to control your chronic pain. Talk with your doctor, then start to control the pain and increase your activities. While it may be unrealistic to expect total pain relief, you can expect to get around in reasonable comfort and do more of the things you want to do. As you manage and win with your chronic pain, you can be more active and enjoy life more.

Let's look again at a few of the most common causes of chronic pain and see what steps actually work to control them.

The most common causes are: chronic back pain, chronic headache pain, chronic jaw pain, cancer pain, and nerve pain.

CHRONIC BACK PAIN

Chronic back pain was discussed on p. 30. If your back pain has been troubling you for months or years, it is time for you to get some relief. The basic medical treatment program for back pain is not complicated but it is important for three reasons:

1. *Most* people do get at least some degree of *pain relief* with only these steps.

2. *Almost all* find that their activity levels can increase.

3. This basic treatment program will increase the chance that the other methods of pain control used *will be successful.*

It is important to remember that with the basic medical treatment program, it is the entire program that gives success, not just one part of the treatment.

Sharon D., a twenty-six-year-old office manager, began the basic treatment program for chronic back pain after an injury. The problem was that Sharon did only a part of the treatment program—the medication and moist heat—saying that she didn't have time to do the exercises or walking. After three months, Sharon felt only slightly improved pain. *If* she had done the entire basic treatment program, including moist heat, exercise, medications, and rest, she would have maximized her pain relief.

Another chronic back pain sufferer, Allan, chose only to take the medication prescribed for relief. He could not understand why he still had pain four months later when he came back to the clinic for an appointment.

After starting the daily exercise program and moist heat, Allan began to feel pain relief and more energy in less than three weeks. *If* he had undergone the program in its entirety when he was diagnosed with the chronic pain, he would probably have experienced greater mobility and less pain.

After months or years of back pain, it is time for you to get relief. The basic treatment program for chronic back pain begins with moist heat and exercises. Let's review the ways that are easiest and most effective to use moist heat.

Moist Heat

You may have tried some form of heating pad at times and found little relief. We suggest that moist heat be used twice daily for ten to twenty minutes on the back, and it should be used *every day without fail.* The most effective and easiest forms of moist heat are a warm shower, hot bath, whirlpool, or heated swimming pool (see figure 3.1). The purpose of moist heat is to help relax the tense muscles, to help decrease the inflammation in the soft tissues of the back, and to relieve pain.

For example, it is easy to put a chair or stool in the shower with rubber tips on the legs for safety. Then let the warm shower hit the back. If you have a whirlpool bath, use it twice daily. Or you may alternate the whirlpool and shower to see which is more effective. A warm bath may work as well, but with chronic pain, it may be difficult to sit or lie down and then get up from the tub. A portable whirlpool for your bathtub may be effective.

If you are not able to use the shower, whirlpool, or bathtub, then warm, moist towels may work. Simply place the moist towels on your back for a few minutes, exchanging them for warm ones when they cool off. Another choice is to use hot packs that can be purchased at a medical supply store. These must be heated in hot water, then wrapped in a towel and placed on the back. Some available packs can be warmed in microwave ovens. These may be easier to use, but don't allow them to get too hot to touch.

A moist heating pad may be effective, especially after improvement in pain from one of the other forms of moist heat. Be sure you use a heating pad designed for moisture. To avoid electrical shock, read the manufacturer's directions before you add moist towels or pads to a heating pad.

Choose the form of moist heat that works best for you, and consider its convenience. Then plan to use this form of moist heat regularly, twice daily, every day. You may find improvement in pain quickly that lasts for a few minutes or hours, but be prepared not to notice a major improvement at first. It takes time.

Figure 3.1. Helpful forms of moist heat for chronic pain

- Heated swimming pool

- Warm whirlpool or hot tub

- Warm shower

- Warm bathtub

- Hot packs as a hydrocollator pack

- Warm, moist towel or cloth

- Moist heating pad

Get Moving!

One of the most important parts of treatment of chronic back pain is an exercise program. Most people who suffer with chronic back pain have been through some form of physical therapy and have yet to find relief. But don't give up yet! *Talk to your doctor before you begin an exercise program to be sure it is safe for you.*

When the muscles supporting the spine are too weak, extra stress is put on the spine. Exercise can remedy this by improving the flexibility of the back to make it more limber and by increasing the strength of the back muscles. If the back becomes more flexible and strong, you will likely notice a decrease in the intensity and/or duration of the pain, and improvement in your level of activity. And these are the concrete goals of the treatment for chronic back pain.

The exercise program that helps in chronic back pain is one that can be done at home. One great benefit of a home exercise program is that it costs very little. But more important, home exercises are convenient and can be done twice daily.

Remember: *exercises for chronic back pain must be done twice daily, without fail.*

Most persons find that the most convenient times to exercise are in the morning and in the evening. Back exercises are given in chapter 4. An easy way to begin these exercises is to do just one each of a few exercises and gradually increase until you can do one of every back exercise comfortably. Then increase to two of each exercise, then three, and gradually increase until you can work up to twenty of each exercise in the morning and twenty of each exercise in the evening.

It will take time for these exercises to affect your chronic back pain, perhaps a couple of weeks to a few months, depending upon your needs. This is where the treatment may be difficult because it involves persistence and patience. Do not be disappointed if you can't see results immediately. Just as an athlete takes time to build muscles, it will take time for the exercises to build the muscles of your back. Reach the goal of twenty repetitions of each exercise twice daily, and the benefits will begin to be more noticeable.

If you don't understand these exercises or if they cause unusual pain, stop until you talk to your doctor.

In our clinic we have found that those people whose chronic back pain dramatically improved are usually the ones who could keep up their exercise program. Try not to start and stop your exercise program. A steady program of gradually increasing exercises is the one that will bring results.

Begin a Daily Walking Program

Walking is a vital part of the basic treatment program. Choose a short distance that you can walk easily, so that you feel no worse when you finish than when you started. This may be only a few yards or less. Don't be embarrassed by this! You must start somewhere to make progress with your chronic pain.

Make yourself walk that same distance each day at least one time. Walk at your own comfortable pace. As you become used to walking short distances, try gradually to increase the distance so that every few days you add a few feet or yards to your total. You will be surprised at how quickly the distance increases. Your goal should be to walk up to two miles each day, but there is no hurry to achieve that distance. Take as long as you need to accomplish the goal. Some people with chronic back pain prefer a treadmill that can be used at home so there is no excuse not to exercise on account of the weather, and it can be done any time, twenty-four hours a day. Talk to your doctor before you begin using a treadmill for exercises.

The importance of the back exercises and the walking program cannot be emphasized enough. Those who can continue these exercises on a regular basis have a much better chance of improving their back pain and their range of activity. Unfortunately, those who don't achieve good results usually are not able to maintain a regular exercise and walking program. It is so important to achieve your goal of improved pain and expanded range activity that if you cannot maintain the program, then you should talk to your doctor to see how it can become possible.

Add Medications

After you have developed chronic back pain, you will probably try many available pain medications. Some of the most commonly used pain relievers are listed below.

MEDICATIONS FOR PAIN RELIEF

The preferred pain medications for pain relief include those available over the counter such as acetaminophen, ibuprofen, and aspirin. In low doses, these medications can relieve many types of pain and have few side effects. Follow the directions on the label. Some other medications used for pain include the noncortisone anti-inflammatory drugs, many of which are available by prescription. These also can act as pain relievers. Some of the most common pain medications are listed in table 3.1. Brand name and generic medications are available for each. If you are taking any other medications, check with your doctor before you begin a pain medication.

Table 3.1. Some common over-the-counter pain medications

Trade Name	Generic Name
Advil, Motrin, Others	Ibuprofen
Ascriptin (with Maalox)	Aspirin
Ecotrin, others	Enteric coated aspirin
8-Hour Bayer, Time Release	Aspirin
Emperin	Aspirin
Many generic and store brands	Aspirin
Tylenol, Anacin-3, Datril, Panadol	Acetaminophen
Generic and store brands	Acetaminophen

Noncortisone Anti-Inflammatory Drugs

One of the noncortisone anti-inflammatory drugs (NSAIDs) may offer pain relief without side effects in some cases. These are more often used in many types of arthritis and are available by prescription from your doctor. There are over twenty available, but it is not possible to predict which person will respond to which drug (see table 3.2). Therefore, it is a good idea to try one medication for about two weeks and judge the effect for yourself. If there is improvement, the particular medication can be continued. If one drug is not helpful, then another might be tried. It does not help to take one of these medications for months at a time, in the hope that it will eventually help. Combining more than one of these drugs is not recommended, since it is unlikely to enhance relief and could increase the chance of side effects. Weigh the benefits of the drug, then decide which medication gives the best relief. Your doctor can tell you if these drugs might be helpful in your own case.

If these drugs give relief, they are quite useful for pain because they are not habit-forming. Although most patients have no side effects from the NSAIDs, each person is different. When side effects do occur, the most common are upset stomach, indigestion, or abdominal pain. In case of these or any other unexplained reactions, you should discontinue the medication until you talk to your doctor.

Table 3.2. Some common noncortisone anti-inflammatory drugs

Trade Name	Generic Name
Advil	Ibuprofen
Anaprox	Naproxyn
Ansaid	Flurbiprofen
Aspirin Products	Aspirin
Clinoril	Sulindac
Daypro	Oxaprozin
Disalcid	Salsalate
Dolobid	Diflunisal
Feldene	Piroxicam
Indocin	Indomethacin

Table 3.2 (cont.)

Trade Name	Generic Name
Lodine	Etodolac
Magan	Magnesium salicylate
Meclomen	Meclofenamate
Nalfon	Fenoprofen
Naprosyn	Naproxyn
Orudis	Ketoprofen
Oruvail	Ketoprofen slow release
Relafen	Nabumetone
Salflex	Salsalate
Tolectin	Tolmetin
Trilisate	Choline magnesium trisalicylate
Voltaren	Diclofenac
Zorprin	Zero-order release aspirin

These drugs may be taken over a long period of time if they give relief and if no side effects occur. You still must watch for side effects as long as you take them. Watch especially for any upset stomach, since peptic ulcer disease can result from their extended use.

If your take these drugs, you need to have a blood test taken every few months to check for side effects. About one percent of those who take these medications for six months or longer may have blood in their stool, so watch out for dark, sticky bowel movements. If you have any questions, talk to your doctor before you continue to take the medications. The most common side effects of this group of medications are listed in table 3.3.

**Table 3.3. Some of the most common side effects
of noncortisone anti-inflammatory drugs**

Indigestion

Heartburn

Abdominal pain

Gastritis

Peptic ulcer

Intestinal bleeding

Diarrhea

Constipation

Rash

Itching

Anemia (lower hemoglobin)

Decreased platelet effect (can affect bleeding)

Changes in the effect of other medication

Sodium retention with edema (swelling)

Increased blood pressure (hypertension)

Possible abnormal liver tests (blood tests)

Possible renal (kidney) failure

Asthma in those allergic

Mouth ulcers

Palpitations

Dizziness

Ringing in the ears (tinnitus)

Sleepiness

Occasional blurred vision

Headaches

Table 3.3 (cont.)

Confusion

Impaired thinking (uncommon, but occurs at times in older patients)

Difficulty in sleeping

Depression

Fatigue

Lowered white cells in blood count

Diminished effect of diuretics

Possible interference with other medications being taken

Sun sensitivity

Meningitis-like illness (rare)

Other individual allergic or unusual reactions.

Narcotics

The stronger pain medications are narcotic drugs. Since these can be habit-forming, they are not desirable for regular use when the pain is long lasting. Narcotics may also cause some drowsiness and may make those who take them less alert. Propxyphene and codeine are probably the most commonly used narcotics for pain.

It is important to ensure when these medications are used for chronic back pain, that the pain is getting better and that your activity level is improving. There is no real advantage in simply killing the pain and being inactive! Some of the most common narcotic drugs are listed in table 3.4.

Table 3.4. Some of the commonly used narcotic drugs

Trade Name	*Generic Name*
Darvon	Propoxyphene
Darvocet, others	Propoxyphene with acetaminophen
Darvon Compound	Propoxyphene with aspirin
Talacen	Pentazocine with acetaminophen
Talwin	Pentazocine
Tylenol #3, Phenaphen #3, other	Codeine
Tylox, Percocet, Roxicet, other	Oxycodone
Vicodin, Lortab, Lorcet, others	Hydrocodone

Other Medications Available

Antidepressants

Other medications can help chronic back pain without the risk of narcotic addiction. For some, relief has been found in a group of medications used for treatment of depression. Although depression can occur in cases of chronic pain, many persons who are not depressed still experience good relief from pain with very small doses of these medications—doses that are usually too small to greatly affect depression. The side effects are usually minimal when low doses are used, but there may be some dryness of mouth, constipation, or drowsiness. When it is given at bedtime, the drowsiness caused by the drug may actually be beneficial if there is no lingering sleepiness the next day. These antidepressants do not usually upset the stomach. They can cause difficulty in urination, so talk with your doctor before starting one of these medications.

As with other medications, you may need to try several different types to see which gives you the best relief. A drug's beneficial effect on pain can usually be felt within two weeks. If there is no improvement, the dose could be increased or another medication of this group could be tried. Some of the most common of these antidepressants and the most common side effects are listed in table 3.5.

**Table 3.5. Some of the most commonly used antidepressant
type medications for pain**

Trade Name	Generic Name
Elavil	Amitriptyline
Norpramin	Desipramine
Pamelor	Nortriptyline
Sinequan	Doxepin
Tofranil	Impramine
Paxil	Paroxetine

Anticonvulsants

Another group of medications, the anticonvulsants, are those used to treat seizures (epilepsy). Some of the most common ones are listed in table 3.6. For some pain sufferers, a trial of one of these may be helpful, but side effects can occur, drowsiness and depression being the most prevalent. Ask your doctor to guide you.

**Table 3.6. Some of the most commonly used anticonvulsant
medications for chronic pain**

Trade Name	Generic Name
Tegretol	Carbamazepine
Dilantin	Phenytoin

Tranquilizers

Tranquilizers are prescription medications which seem appealing for their help in relieving the anxiety of chronic back pain and for helping sufferers sleep at night. However, they can be habit-forming, and the positive effect may be lost after a period of time. They do not often help a person with chronic back pain to be more active; commonly they reduce activity. Your doctor can assist you in deciding whether you ought to take them. Some of the most common tranquilizers are diazepam (Valium), chlorodiazepoxide (Librium), and lorezepam (Ativan).

Muscle Relaxants

Muscle relaxants can be helpful in relieving chronic back pain when a muscle spasm is the culprit. Relaxants can be used as needed if they give good pain relief, an increase in activity with pain relief, and if there is not too much drowsiness from the medication. The most commonly used muscle relaxants are given in table 3.7. These are available by prescription from your doctor.

Table 3.7. Some of the commonly used muscle relaxants for chronic pain

Trade Name	Generic Name
Flexeril	Cyclobenzaprine
Parafon Forte	Chlorzoxazone
Robaxin	Methocarbamol
Skelaxin	Metaxalone
Soma	Carisoprodol

Local Injections

Local injections can be helpful in relieving chronic back pain when there are localized areas of pain (trigger points). These injections often use a local anesthetic that can be combined with a low dose of a cortisone derivative. There is often relief of pain from the localized trigger point and other areas of pain caused by the trigger points. Pain improves within a few days, with relief often lasting for weeks at a time. This treatment is especially good when there are one or two trigger points causing major pain and limitation. Also, if there is improvement in many areas but one or two painful areas remain, then local injection can be very helpful in achieving overall pain control.

There are usually no serious side effects from the use of local injections. The cortisone dose used is usually low and should have little effect on the body, so there should be no significant problems from an occasional local injection of these areas of soft tissue pain.

Combination Treatment with Medications

Depending on the specific causes of the pain, in our clinic, we find that a combination of heat and exercise along with the most effective noncortisone anti-inflammatory drug and one of the above-mentioned antidepressant medications often gives major relief in treating chronic back pain. It does require some trial and error with the medications, however. It is important that you and your doctor patiently try the available medications in each group to be sure you have the best chance for success in pain control and increased levels of activity, since each person is different.

STRESS REDUCTION WITH CHRONIC PAIN

Chronic back pain causes stress in all areas of life, with much stress arising from the pain itself, from effects on the family, loss of income, loss of job, and many other areas (see chapter 7). In recent years it has been found that the control of chronic back pain can be greatly improved with the addition of psychological treatment. In fact, this is an extremely important part of any chronic pain treatment, since results often show major decreases in the amount of pain medication used and increases in the patient's level of activity.

Several areas are important in psychological treatment. Behavior can be adjusted to avoid dependence on bed rest, drugs, and inactivity to ease pain. Other forms of therapy teach patients how to manage their pain by changing the way they cope with it. Researchers have found that depression is common in patients who suffer with chronic back pain; treatment of the depression can improve the results of pain control.

When these areas of treatment are added to the medical treatment programs, improvement does occur. People learn that they can regain control of their pain and increase their range of activity. For example, the chances of returning to work after being out of work from back pain for more than six months are extremely low. But one center found that with the inclusion of psychological treatment, *almost 30 percent of those who had been out of work for over two and a half years returned to work!* Chapter 7 offers specific steps you can take to enable you to help control stress and benefit from some psychological evaluation.

Many chronic pain sufferers feel worried or embarrassed about psychological evaluation or treatment. This does *not* mean that the pain is "in your head." This is a standard part of the treatment plan that works. Psychologists and psychiatrists happen to be those specialists qualified in this part of treatment for chronic pain.

MASSAGE

Gentle rubbing of the muscles, tendons, and other soft tissues can improve relaxation and bring comfort to those who experience chronic back pain. The period of comfort that occurs after a massage may last for hours. If massage significantly benefits your back pain, we suggest you consider finding a licensed professional massage therapist or physical therapist to be sure massage is done properly to achieve its full effect. It can be repeated as often as needed.

MANIPULATION

Spinal manipulation for back pain is a very old technique that led to the development of chiropractic and osteopathy. Spinal manipulation, also called spinal adjustment, has the goal of pain relief by increasing the mobility of the spinal bones (vertebrae) that have become restricted in movement or out of proper position.

Manipulation of the spine involves techniques by using the hands to attempt to restore more normal mobility to the joints and reduce pain. Manipulations involve either repeated motions of gentle stretching and pressure or high velocity thrust movements to the spine. It is hoped that manipulation improves mobility, reduces inflammation, and improves relaxation of the surrounding muscles.

Relief in back pain after manipulation may be immediate or delayed. If pain does not improve or becomes worse, then other methods of pain relief should be used. Manipulation is not done when there is a possibility of infection, fracture of a bone, cancer, or severe arthritis in the spine.

Manipulation may be used by your doctor to improve pain relief. Like other methods of treatment, if it helps to control pain and increase activity, it can be continued.

ULTRASOUND

Ultrasound uses sound waves that are applied to the muscles, tendons, and other soft tissues of the back. This may help relaxation, decrease inflammation, and improve back pain. It is usually more effective and more commonly used in acute back pain and other similar situations than in chronic pain. It can be done properly by your physical therapist and continued if it gives relief.

TRANSCUTANEOUS ELECTRICAL NERVE STIMULATION (TENS)

This technique uses electrical stimulation for pain relief. TENS has been used to relieve pain from many different causes. The idea is that electrical impulses sent to certain nerves block the messages of pain being sent by other nerves from the painful area. It might also cause the release of endorphins, which are natural pain relievers produced by the body.

Back pain sufferers wear the stimulator and battery, usually on their belts (see figure 3.2). Electrical wires from the stimulator are attached to electrodes placed on the skin with an adhesive patch at the painful area. The electrodes are placed in the area of pain but may need to be tried at different locations to get the best relief.

The TENS unit can be controlled by the pain sufferer and can be used continuously or only as needed for the pain. Usually there will be a trial of about one month to see the effect on pain.

BRACES

Braces and other supports are *not* recommended for constant use for most persons with chronic back pain. These limit movement of the spine, which may give some temporary relief, but they may also allow the muscles of the back to become weaker, thus limiting flexibility. If used when the pain is severe, they should then be removed twice daily for exercises unless your doctor tells you otherwise.

STILL NO RELIEF?

What if there is still not enough pain relief of back pain and insufficient range of activity? You should nevertheless continue the twice-daily moist heat and exercises, the walking, and your efforts to find the most effective combination of medications. In addition, there are other measures, such as nerve blocks, that may offer relief from pain. These treatments

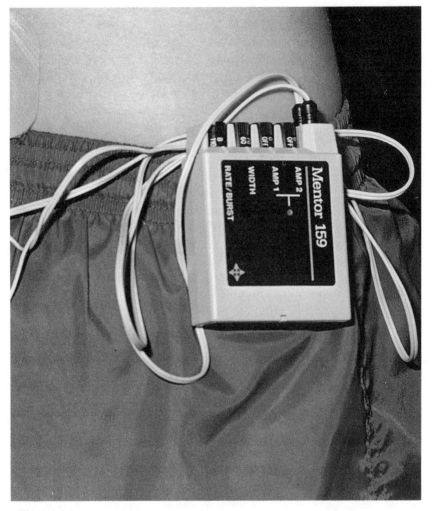

Figure 3.2. The TENS unit uses electrical stimulation for pain relief.

become more expensive and require more procedures, but are worth it if they give the needed relief.

NERVE BLOCKS

Through injection of medication around a nerve, nerve blocks can give relief of pain, but they may not be long-lasting for many chronic pain sufferers. If the relief lasts for weeks to months, these injections become more acceptable for repeated use. At times, there can be long-lasting improvement in pain after a nerve block.

Nerve blocks can also be used to see what portion of the pain is relieved. If there is excellent relief of pain, then a more permanent type of nerve block attempt, as that discussed on p. 140, may be considered. If nerve blocks along with the other steps discussed give no relief, it may be a good idea to consider further treatment as discussed in chapter 5 or evaluation in a comprehensive pain clinic (see p. 150).

BEGINNING TREATMENT FOR OSTEOPOROSIS

Osteoporosis, as a cause of chronic pain, is usually discovered after there has been a fracture in the spine or some other bone. If a bone density test is done, then, of course, osteoporosis may be detected earlier. Once the diagnosis is made, the treatment plan is started to try to prevent the next fracture. Newer medications allow for the possibility of increasing the strength of the bones and, if all goes well, prevention of future fractures.

Add Exercises

Add a regular exercise program for the back. Start slowly and gradually with the back exercises outlined in chapter 4, doing only one or two of an exercise each morning and evening. You will get the best results if you are shown how to do the back exercises correctly by a physical therapist. Then continue twice daily exercises every day, without fail.

Make yourself keep up the exercises on both good days and bad days. Gradually increase from one or two to three, then four, and as you are able, increase all the way up to twenty of each exercise twice each day. This may take weeks or months to accomplish, but keep trying. Don't increase *too* quickly: let yourself feel comfortable at one level first, then move on. It is more important to make the exercise program long-lasting than to increase the number of repetitions too quickly.

The back exercises make the spine more flexible and limber. They also increase the strength of the muscles that support the spine. With more strength and support the back will work better: your activity can increase, but it will take from a few weeks to a few months to see any major effect.

Include a Walking Program

A walking program like the one we already discussed is very important for treating osteoporosis and preventing future fractures. Walking and other activities that bear weight on the bones help to stimulate them to become stronger. Don't forget to pick a short distance and walk it every day, even if only a few yards. Then gradually increase the distance as you can. You'll be surprised how quickly you are able to increase your distance.

We saw a woman with osteoporosis and fractures in the spine who required treatment in the hospital because of several fractures and severe back pain. After following the treatment program, two months later she was able to walk over one mile each day. As her walking program improved, she was able to resume other daily activities, including her work as a volunteer in a child care center.

Add 1500 mg of Calcium Each Day

Be sure to consume enough calcium each day. The goal should be about a total of 1500 mg of calcium daily combined from your diet and supplements. An easy way to manage this is to calculate roughly about how much calcium is in your average day's diet using high calcium foods given in table 3.8. Then supplement this amount with calcium available at drug stores and health food stores. A list of common calcium supplements is given in table 3.9. The total should equal about 1500 mg. For example, if your calcium intake from food is about 900 mg each day, you need about 600 mg of calcium supplement. This is about three tablets of 200 mg or the equivalent (see list of calcium supplements).

It is not necessary to take higher amounts. There are very few side effects from this amount of calcium. If you have kidney stones (deposits of calcium), check with your doctor first, since you may need to modify this amount. There are tests that can determine if you are likely to develop kidney stones after you increase your intake of calcium.

Table 3.8. Common foods with high calcium content

Food	Amount	Calcium Content
Beans, baked	1 cup	150 mg
Beans, black	1 cup	250
Broccoli	1 cup	145
Cheese, American	1 slice	200
Cheddar cheese	1 cup	845
Cottage cheese	1 cup	140
Reduced calorie, low-fat cheese	1 oz.	200
Chocolate milk, 1% milkfat	8 oz.	300
Evaporated condensed milk	8 oz.	800
Evaporated skim milk	8 oz.	500–600
Ice cream	1 cup	175–270
Kale	1 cup	205
Milk, homogenized cow's milk	8 oz.	500
Milk, cow's, skim	8 oz.	300
Monterey cheese	1 oz.	200
Okra, steamed	1 cup	150
Salmon	8 medium	350–450
Spinach, steamed	1 cup	170
Sweet potato, canned	1 cup	85
Turnip greens	1 cup	270
Yogurt	8 oz.	300
Frozen	6 oz.	150

Table 3.9. Commonly used over-the-counter calcium supplements

Name	Type of Calcium	Actual Amount of Calcium
Tums tablets	calcium carbonate	200 mg/tablet
Tums E-X tablets	calcium carbonate	300 mg/tablet
Digel tablets	calcium carbonate	112 mg/tablet
Biocal calcium supplement tablets	calcium carbonate	500 mg/tablet
Dorcal children's liquid supplement	glubionate calcium	115 mg/tsp.
Os-Cal 500 tablets	oyster shell	500 mg/tablet
Titralac tablets	calcium carbonate	168 mg/tablet

Include Vitamin D in Your Diet

Since vitamin D helps the body absorb calcium from the intestine, be sure you have enough vitamin D through your diet or by way of supplements. The recommended daily amount is 400–800 units daily, which can be taken from food sources as given in table 3.10. Most multivitamins contain 400 units of vitamin D, which is a source easily available over the counter (see table 3.11).

Table 3.10. Some common sources of vitamin D in food

Food	Serving Size	Vitamin D (IU)
Cereals		
Bran Flakes	¾ cup	100
Raisin Bran	¾ cup	100
Eel, smoked	3½ oz.	6400
Egg	1 medium	27
Egg substitute	¼ cup	26
Cod-liver oil	2 tsp.	800
Herring	3 oz.	840
Margarine	1 tbsp.	45
Sardines, canned in oil	3½ oz.	300
Salmon (Atlantic) canned	3½ oz.	500
Tuna	2 oz.	168
Milk, fortified	1 cup	100
Milk, evaporated, canned	½ cup	44

Table 3.11. Some commonly used calcium with vitamin D supplements

Name	Actual Amount of Calcium	Amount of Vitamin D
Calcet tablets	240 mg/tablet	100 IU
	152 mg/tablet	
Dical-D	350 mg	399 IU
Dical-D	464 mg	400 IU
Os-Cal 250 + D	250 mg/tablet	125 IU

Estrogen Is Effective in Preventing Bone Loss

Estrogen, the female hormone, is used to treat osteoporosis. Especially around the time of menopause, estrogen can be very effective in preventing bone deterioration. There is evidence that it may also increase the rate of bone formation. This treatment is available for women who have reached menopause or who have had surgery to remove the ovaries, which produce the body's own estrogen. The dose required to be effective in osteoporosis is at least 0.625 mg of conjugated estrogen daily. Some physicians may also combine another female hormone, progesterone, in low doses to try to make the total hormone replacement as natural as possible.

There are some possible side effects of estrogen treatment. This treatment may not be advisable if there has been breast cancer, breast cysts, hypertension, blood clots, or other medical problems. Your doctor can help you decide whether the benefits outweigh the risks of estrogen treatment in your own situation.

Smoking

If you smoke cigarettes, stopping can reduce your risk of osteoporosis, perhaps by up to one-half. Avoid heavy alcohol use because it can make osteoporosis worsen.

Medications

Some medications can cause increased osteoporosis. Most common are prednisone and other cortisone derivatives. When these are used, try to keep them at the lowest possible dose for the shortest length of time. Some medical problems and their treatments can increase the risk of osteoporosis, such as emphysema, chronic bronchitis, and rheumatoid arthritis. These problems should be controlled as much as possible but with special attention given to their effects on osteoporosis.

Other Medications to Treat Osteoporosis

Other medications available by prescription from your doctor may actually help increase the bone density. Calcitonin is available by injection, usually two to seven times weekly. It is somewhat inconvenient because it requires injections which can increase bone density.

Another group of medicines is becoming available to treat osteoporosis. Etidronate is a tablet that is taken for two weeks about four times a year. Newer types of this group of medications called bisphosphonates are now being developed and tested. Other newer medicines are also in research stages now, so try to keep informed.

Fluoride has been used for years for osteoporosis. It has some limitations in dose and it does have possible side effects: nausea, diarrhea, or other intestinal symptoms. There is also some controversy as to whether fluoride can actually lower the number of fractures even though it may make the bone density increase.

Researchers will likely provide more information in the future about fluoride, bisphosphonates, and other new treatments. The main point now is to be aware that *there is treatment available that has a good chance of increasing bone density and reducing future fractures.*

Bone density can be measured at yearly intervals to determine the effect of the treatment on the bones and whether there has been an increase in the bone density (see figure 3.3).

THE CHRONIC PAIN OF ARTHRITIS

It is important to know exactly what types of arthritis are causing your pain. As discussed in chapter 2, there are over one hundred types of arthritis. The treatment may be different for many forms of the disease. For example, gout is a form of arthritis that can cause chronic pain. But with simple medication, gout can be completely controlled. Other forms of arthritis also have excellent treatment available.

You may very well have more than one type of arthritis at the same time. For example, you may have had osteoarthritis for years in the knees, hips, or back. If there is worsening of pain and stiffness in the joints, it is possible that a second type of arthritis has developed. We see patients who develop rheumatoid arthritis or gout as a second type of arthritis. The second arthritis may in fact be the main cause of pain, and there could well be better treatment available.

Talk with your doctor to determine what type(s) of arthritis you must deal with. You may choose to be seen by a rheumatologist, i.e., a physician who specializes in treating arthritis.

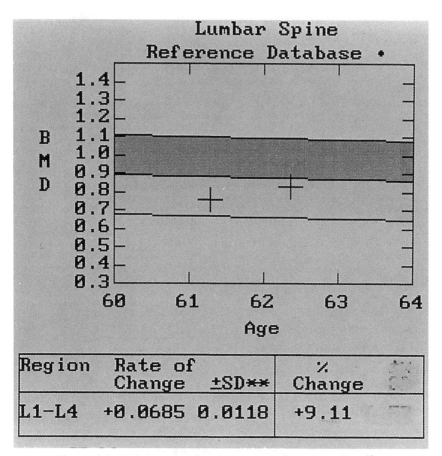

Figure 3.3. A bone density report can show you the effect
of treatment for osteoporosis.

BEGIN TREATMENT FOR PAIN RELIEF

Once the diagnosis of arthritis is final, begin a basic treatment program. This can be done at home.

Start with Moist Heat

One of the most successful approaches in our clinic is the use of a warm shower or bathtub.

Put a skid-proof chair or stool in the shower and let the warm shower run on the painful areas for ten to fifteen minutes each morning and each evening. The moist heat will help relax the painful muscles, help decrease joint inflammation, and help increase flexibility to make you more limber.

The warm bathtub can also be used provided you can get in and out comfortably. It isn't necessary to have the water very hot, just warm enough so it is comfortable. As we've seen, for some the bathtub may be difficult because it may be too painful to get in and out, particularly when there is arthritis in the knees and hips. In these cases we recommend using the shower or a chair or stool in the bathtub.

Another form of moist heat is a whirlpool bath. This is effective, since it can add some effect of massage to the warm water. If you have one available, it may be the most effective. Many patients in our clinic tell us this gives the best relief.

If these forms of moist heat are not available or inconvenient, then you can use warm moist towels or hot packs. Apply the moist towels to the painful joints for about fifteen minutes twice daily. The hot packs can be heated, then wrapped in towels and placed around the joints for fifteen minutes twice daily.

Some hot packs are available that can be heated in a microwave oven, which may make them more convenient. Water can also be warmed in a microwave oven for the moist towels. Be careful when using the microwave as the temperature can rapidly become very hot. Always test the temperature of the moist towel or hot pack before applying these to your skin.

A heated swimming pool is another effective way to use moist heat. When the arthritis pain is not localized but all over, this is especially useful. You can use the pool when available and then use one of the other forms of heat at other times, twice daily.

Choose the form of moist heat that is most effective and easiest for you. We suggest that you find a method that offers relief as well as convenience. Otherwise it will be hard to continue it regularly. The benefits of the moist heat in arthritis pain will be felt best when used twice daily.

When arthritis pain affects the hands, a form of heat is available which may be especially effective for relief. A warm mixture of paraffin and mineral oil is an excellent way to deliver heat to the hands and to give relief from arthritis pain. A small portable unit can be used at home very easily, twice daily. For those whose arthritis affects the hands, this often gives excellent relief.

Other forms of heat include heating pads. A moist heating pad may give some relief, especially after there has been improvement in arthritis pain. Usually at first, the other forms of heat will be more effective. But the heating pad is convenient and, if it gives relief, that's what counts.

Ice Can Relieve Pain

Ice has been used in some cases to relieve arthritis. Although most patients prefer the effects of heat, some gain relief with ice packs or even alternating periods of ice and heat. When ice is used it should be placed in a plastic bag around the joint. To avoid injury, do not place ice directly on the skin. It can be used for periods of about ten minutes and repeated two or three times daily.

EXERCISE FOR MOBILITY AND PAIN CONTROL

Along with the moist heat, it is extremely important to add exercises for the joints affected by arthritis. The exercises in chapter 4 are recommended to make the joints more flexible and limber. They also build up the strength of the muscles that support the joints. With more support, there is a better chance for improvement in pain and stiffness. If the muscles are not strong, then movement will be more difficult, even without arthritis!

We suggest that exercises be done simultaneously with use of the moist heat: this means in the shower, bathtub, or whirlpool, or while hot packs are applied to the joints. This makes the exercises easier and more effective. Start with one of each exercise in the morning session and one in the evening session. Then gradually increase the repetitions until the goal of twenty repetitions, twice daily, is reached. You may take as long as needed gradually to increase to twenty repetitions. If your pain does not lessen, then stop until you talk to your doctor. If you don't understand the exercises, let your doctor or physical therapist help you.

Exercises may be the most important part of the treatment for arthritis, and at times they may be more effective than medication. If your goal is to take less medication (or none at all), then take the time to do the exercises, twice daily. We spend much time in our clinic explaining and emphasizing the value of these exercises. Most patients tell us that they experience more pain and simply don't feel as well if they miss their exercises.

Rest to Control Fatigue

In arthritis, tiredness and fatigue may be a major problem in addition to the pain. The cause of such fatigue is not known, but is probably related to the inflammation of arthritis. Fatigue can make all daily activities harder to complete. When fatigue is severe, try to have a rest period late in the morning and late in the afternoon. It is not necessary to sleep; you can just watch TV or listen to music.

Simply lie down or relax for ten minutes. Many people lie on a couch in their office, then continue to work after the rest time. These periods of rest can help the fatigue of arthritis and may make the remainder of your day and evening more enjoyable. Then as your arthritis improves, these rest times can be shortened or even stopped altogether.

ARTHRITIS MEDICATIONS

When arthritis pain is *not* controlled by low doses of medications available over the counter, such as ibuprofen, acetaminophen, or aspirin, then there are other medications your doctor can prescribe that may help.

The most commonly used arthritis medications are intended to relieve pain, swelling, and stiffness caused by inflammation in and around the joints. These anti-inflammatory drugs are of two main types. The most common noncortisone anti-inflammatory drugs have already been listed in table 3.2. The cortisone-type drugs are the strongest anti-inflammatory drugs and are reserved for more severe cases because of the possibility of more side effects.

Table 3.12. Some commonly used cortisone-type drugs for chronic pain

Trade Name	*Generic Name*
Deltasone, Metacortin, Orasone	prednisone
Medrol	methylprednisolone
Aristocort	triamcinolone
Decadron, Hexadrol, Kenalog	dexamethasone
Celestone	betamethasone

Nonsteroid Anti-Inflammatory Medications

There is no definite way to predict which of the nonsteroid (noncortisone) anti-inflammatory drugs (NSAIDs) will work in each person. It is a good idea to try one for about two weeks and judge the effect. If there is improvement in pain and stiffness, then it can be continued. If not, then try another until you find the one that works best.

Most people find a drug that works without side effects. If you can't tell any difference, then the drug you're taking probably is not helping enough to warrant its continued use.

Side effects with such drugs are not unusual. If you do experience side effects, the most common are likely to be nausea, upset stomach, or abdominal pain. The other common potential side effects are listed on p. 73. As long as you take these medications you should watch closely for any side effects, and, if need be, discontinue use of the drugs if you experience any unexplained new side effects.

These drugs can be taken safely over months to years if discernible side effects don't occur and if blood tests are conducted every few months for safety. About one percent of those who take these medications for six months or longer may have bloody stool, so you should watch for any dark, sticky bowel movements and for blood in the stool.

Remember: the fewer medications you take the better. The way to be able to reduce the need for these and other medications for the chronic pain of arthritis is to keep up a regular program of moist heat and exercises in addition to medication.

Cortisone-Type Medications

The cortisone-type medications are used in low doses in more severe cases of arthritis and when there is internal organ disease present in some types of the disease. For example, inflammation around the heart (pericarditis) or kidney in some types of arthritis is often treated with the cortisone-type drugs. Your doctor can guide you. These can also be used in local injections in the joints and can give very good relief in a specific joint without effecting other areas. When one joint is much more severely effected than others, cortisone-type medication can be helpful in allowing more activity and gaining additional comfort. The chance of side effects from the local injection is low.

If you try all the available anti-inflammatory medications and still find no relief, there are other possibilities for treatment. First, be sure about the diagnosis of arthritis and whether a second type of arthritis may be present. If so, then different treatments may be available.

Suppressive Medications

For rheumatoid arthritis and other severe arthritis conditions there is another group of medications that may suppress the symptoms at a more basic level. They may give better control of the pain, swelling, stiffness, and fatigue of arthritis. Many give up to an 80 percent chance of improvement. But these medications are slower-acting, usually taking about three months to show a noticeable effect. They also have some possible side effects, although these are usually easy to control. When the medications are taken, they must be monitored by your doctor through regular lab testing. Some of the most commonly used of this group of medications are listed in table 3.13.

SURGERY CAN HELP

If adequate relief has still not been achieved after using heat, exercises, and a full regime of available medications, then it may be necessary to consider surgery to relieve the arthritis. Surgery can be of help when the pain is constant and severe or when use of the joint has become very limited by the arthritis despite treatment. For example, in osteo-arthritis the cartilage of the knee or hip can be so damaged the treatments already discussed, including heat, exercise, and medication, do not give enough relief (see figure 3.4); or in rheumatoid arthritis there may be

Table 3.13. Some commonly used suppressive medications

Trade Name	*Generic Name*
Gold Compounds	
Ridaura (capsule)	auranofin
Myochrisine (injection)	gold sodium thiomalate
Solgonal (injection)	gold aurothioglucose
Rheumatrex (tablets & injection)	methotrexate
Plaquenil (tablets)	hydroxychloroquine
Imuran (tablets)	azathioprine
Depen (tablets)	penicillamine
Cuprimine (capsules)	penicillamine
Azulfidine	sulfasalazine

so much swelling and thickening of the joint lining that the heat, exercises, and medications already discussed may have no effect.

Joint Replacement and Arthroscopy

The types of most frequently performed arthritis surgery are total joint replacement and arthroscopy. Total joint replacement is a procedure used in osteoarthritis and rheumatoid arthritis. It works especially well in the hip and knee. An artificial joint is inserted, which usually gives excellent results in diminishing the pain, and allows for a much wider range of activity.

In arthroscopy, a light is inserted into the joint to view it directly. Damaged cartilage in the joint, damaged ligaments, and other problems can be discovered. The abnormality may be able to be repaired or corrected at the same time. Arthroscopy requires much less recovery time than other more involved types of surgery.

There are other types of surgery available in the treatment of arthritis; for example, in the case of rheumatoid arthritis, removal of the swollen and painful lining of the joint, such as the knee joint. This is usually done before extensive joint destruction occurs. This procedure may provide some pain relief in the affected knee for three to five years. We recommend a complete consultation with your doctor or orthopedic surgeon, who specializes in joint and bone surgery.

HEADACHES

The treatment of chronic headache pain can begin after proper diagnosis to be sure no other serious underlying problem is present. Another disease or condition which can cause headaches may be able to be treated specifically.

Muscle Contraction Headache

For this most frequent type of chronic headache pain, a regular program of neck, back, and shoulder exercises is recommended. These exercises keep the muscles of the neck flexible and strong. Many persons find improvement in their headaches and neck pain as they see improvement in muscle strength. (These exercises are listed in chapter 4.)

Pain medications available over the counter may help relieve discomfort. These include acetaminophen, ibuprofen, and aspirin.

As we have learned, a group of antidepressant medications has been used with some effect in chronic back pain and chronic neck pain and the headaches these conditions cause, especially when the headaches occur daily or even several times a day. These anti-depressant-type medications are listed in table 3.5.

Your doctor may need to try a few different medications for one to two weeks at a time to find the one most effective for your headaches. Depression can also accompany these muscle contraction headaches; but improvement in the headaches can occur when these medications are used, with or without improvement in the depression. Muscle relaxants are acceptable for use if they give relief.

Since stress is often present with muscle contraction headaches; when the headaches become chronic it is helpful to consider psychological evaluation and instruction in stress management techniques. These are simple techniques easily taught so that pain sufferers can manage stress more effectively. (See the relaxation response in chapter 5 for additional assistance with stress reduction.)

Headaches Due to Arthritis in the Neck

For headaches arising from arthritis in the neck, the first step is to obtain specific treatment for the type of arthritis present. Talk with your doctor and begin a basic treatment program. (See p. 89.) This usually includes twice-daily moist heat, such as a shower or warm towels. Exercises for the neck and back are very important in the treatment

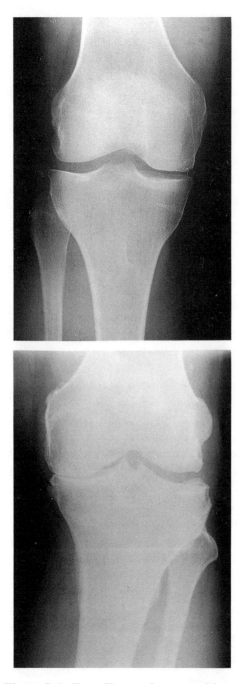

**Figure 3.4. Top: X-ray of a normal knee
Bottom: X-ray of a knee with arthritis**

of arthritis in the neck. (See the exercises in chapter 4.) Try to work up to twenty repetitions twice daily for each exercise. Remember to allow a few weeks to two months to notice improvement.

Medications are available, depending on the type of arthritis thought to cause the headache. Most people find some combination of heat, exercise, and medication brings the longest and most significant relief.

A soft cervical collar available at drug stores or medical supply stores may be used during periods of more severe pain from arthritis in the neck. These are worn when the pain is severe and may be removed when the pain subsides. They should not be worn consistently without instruction by your doctor.

Traction (see p. 101), can be used at times for relief of head and neck pain due to osteoarthritis. Check with your doctor first to be sure it is safe.

Vascular Headaches

Medications are available to treat migraine headache, both the occasional short-term acute headache and those which are more frequent (more than weekly) or limiting in their intensity. These were listed on p. 70. Migraine headache medications need to be prescribed by your physician because they have potentially serious side effects and must be used very carefully.

The new drug sumatriptan (Imitrex) is an injection that will not prevent migraines, but is effective for the pain of migraine in most patients. Serotonin (a body enzyme) appears to reduce headache by raising the pain threshold. The drug sumatriptan works on serotonin release instead of blood vessel spasm and may provide relief in less than twenty minutes as it alleviates the nausea, head pain, and light sensitivity.

Some persons are sensitive to certain foods that may cause headaches for unknown reasons. A short list would include: coffee, some wines, cheese, monosodium glutamate (MSG), as well as nitrites in foods such as hot dogs and other cured meats. These can aggravate chronic headaches.

For other medical problems that cause headaches, the pain will not subside until the underlying medical difficulty has been treated. Causes include hypertension, infections, sinus diseases, diseases of the eye and ear, and tumors. Your doctor can give you advice and recommend appropriate treatment.

JAW PAIN AND FACIAL PAIN

As we have said, diagnosis of the specific causes of jaw or facial pain is important (see p. 53) since many such causes are treatable. For example, there may be an infection or some underlying dental problem. If no other definite causes are found, then the treatment outlined for soft tissue pain—the common cause of temporomandibular joint (TMJ) syndrome—may help. TMJ syndrome is the most common cause of jaw pain. We recommend a step-by-step approach:

1. If you have dental problems, these should be taken care of by your dentist. These can include loose or poorly fitting dentures or missing teeth. Any imbalance in the way the teeth come together should be addressed and corrected, if possible. This can reduce stress resulting from an abnormal chewing motion.

2. Apply moist heat to the jaw areas just in front of the ear: try a warm, moist cloth for ten to fifteen minutes at least twice daily. This may give temporary relief.

3. Try to *manage the stress* in your life: a little more relaxation can help by lowering the tension in the powerful muscles of the jaw and thus decreasing the pressure on the TMJ. The relaxation response in chapter 5 is an excellent way to lower tension and can be learned with a little practice.

4. When there is jaw pain, avoid chewing gum as well as hard or chewy foods such as taffy and tough steak, since these cause much higher pressures in both jaw joints and can increase pain.
When there is TMJ or other jaw pain, it is important to try to *chew food as evenly as possible* on both sides of the mouth; alternate chewing on your left and right side if you can. This helps distribute the pressure equally on the jaw joints and muscles.

5. Your family can help by noticing whether you happen to have a habit of clenching, grinding, or gritting your teeth at night. If you do, you may benefit from a special *dental splint* to wear at night to protect the teeth and take stress off the TMJ. At times a mild sedative at bedtime may be needed for relaxation if other steps do not work.

6. Some *medications* are excellent in reducing the pain around the TMJ. While many must be prescribed, some are available over the counter (e.g, ibuprofen) and give excellent relief.

ARTHRITIS AND JAW PAIN

If you have arthritis in other areas of your body, it can also attack the TMJ just as it would any other joint. If the jaw pain becomes more severe, one of the noncortisone anti-inflammatory drugs listed in table 3.2 may give relief. Your doctor may want you to try one for about two weeks and judge the effect. If there is no improvement, then you may want to try a few different anti-inflammatory drugs.

If there is even more wearing of the joint, followed by deformity from loss of the cartilage coupled with unbearable pain that cannot be relieved by treatment, arthroscopy (see p. 95) may be of some help. Also, MRI (Magnetic Resonance Imaging) can help determine the exact cause of the jaw disorder.

In some cases surgery may be possible to repair or replace the TMJ for pain relief. Surgical treatments are usually reserved until all other treatment options have failed.

If there is continued pain which travels into the temple, jaw, throat, or neck, or if pain spreads to the face, then it may be a sign that the underlying problem is not improving. In this case you should check again with your physician or dentist to see whether any other physical problem could be causing the pain.

CHRONIC NECK PAIN

Chronic Neck Strain

The soft tissues of the neck are the main source of pain in chronic neck strain. The most effective treatment includes twice daily moist heat such as shower or moist towels as outlined on p. 68. The shower and whirlpool work especially well. Moist heat should be used for fifteen to twenty minutes each morning and evening.

In the shower or immediately after, add exercises for the neck, back, and shoulders as shown in chapter 4. Strengthening these muscles can help give more support to the neck.

Gradually increase from one or two of each exercise each morning and evening up to twenty repetitions twice daily. If there is severe pain, stop all exercise until you talk to your doctor. If you experience dizziness, shortness of breath, or other problems with exercise, then talk to your doctor before beginning any exercise.

Medications for the pain of chronic neck strain are commonly taken from two groups listed in tables 3.2 and 3.5. The noncortisone and anti-inflammatory drugs, as discussed on pp. 71–72, often give relief of the pain and stiffness of inflammation from arthritis in the neck. And the group of anti-depressant-type medications may give additional help in pain control.

Finding the most effective medication combination may take time and patience. It is important to isolate the one that gives the best relief of pain without side effects.

Arthritis in the Neck

Pain from arthritis of the neck requires treatment of the underlying arthritic condition. For example, osteoarthritis, the most common type of arthritis in the neck, is best treated with twice daily moist heat with exercises for the neck, back, and shoulders. You should gradually increase the exercises until you can do twenty of each exercise twice daily.

Finding the most effective nonsteroid anti-inflammatory drug which also causes no side effects may take time and patience. Other types of arthritis may have specific treatments available.

Another group of medications used in chronic back pain and chronic headaches may also be very helpful in arthritis of the neck. This group of anti-depressant-type medications is listed in table 3.5. It may take time and trials of a few different drug therapies to see which is the most beneficial. Try to be patient as you go through several medications.

Traction can be used at times, mainly in osteoarthritis involving the neck. A weight on a pulley is attached to a strap under the chin which pulls the head with tension from the chin (see figure 3.5). This may be continued if pain improves. Check with your doctor to see if this is a safe method of treatment for your pain. If it is, you should be given detailed instructions by a physical therapist in the use of traction.

Other problems such as tumors, cancer, and other medical conditions are less common causes of neck pain but certainly require attention. Your doctor can give you advice on the specific treatments needed.

Neck Pain with Pressure on a Nerve

Neck pain can sometimes become severe with pain and numbness traveling down the arm to the hand. This is discussed on p. 58. If the pain and numbness continue despite treatment, then you should consider seeking another medical opinion to decide which of a number of additional tests might provide an answer.

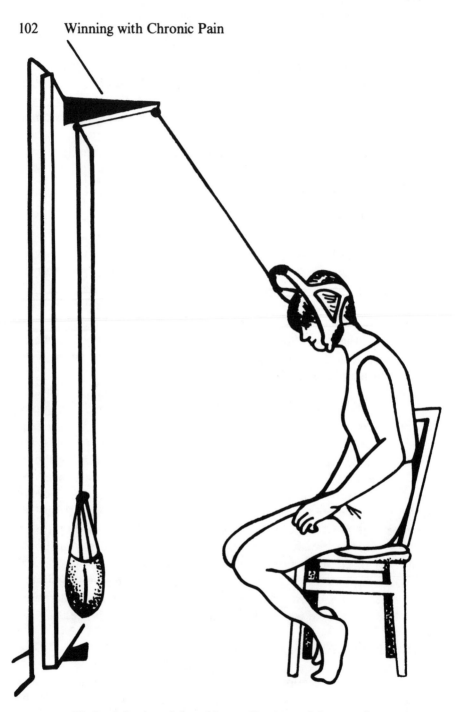

Figure 3.5. A weight with a pulley is used for traction in treatment of chronic neck pain.

Most people do not need surgery even with known pressure on a nerve from a ruptured disc in the neck. But if your pain and numbness are severely limiting or accompanied by muscle weakness, then it is a good idea to consult a neurosurgeon or neurologist. If the diagnosis of ruptured disc is confirmed and no improvement occurs over months of treatment, then surgery may be necessary for relief. Your surgeon can advise you about the benefits and the risks of surgery for the treatment of a ruptured disc in the neck.

CANCER PAIN

Medications are the most common ways to treat the pain of cancer. These include non-narcotic pain medications such as ibuprofen, acetaminophen, and aspirin or one of the noncortisone anti-inflammatory drugs. (These include a large number of medications as shown in table 3.2.) Some choices combine a non-narcotic drug with a narcotic.

Narcotics in Cancer Pain

When narcotics are used regularly, usually over a period of weeks, physical dependence may result. In this situation, withdrawal symptoms occur if the narcotic is suddenly stopped. If the narcotic is gradually decreased, such symptoms can be avoided. Tolerance to the narcotic can develop, wherein higher doses are needed to achieve pain relief. In reality, however, in cancer pain this is not very likely: more often than not, narcotic dosages are lower than needed for pain relief because of fear that addiction might occur. True narcotic addiction is very uncommon when treating chronic pain, especially cancer pain. Frequent requests for drugs may make patients appear to be addicted, but these requests are due more often to lower doses being used than are needed for pain control (see table 3.14).

Each person is different, and the choice of narcotics and the manner in which the narcotic is given to the patient must be tailored to that person. With the large number of narcotics available and the number of ways possible to receive the medication, most patients should be able to achieve pain relief.

Table 3.14. Narcotic drugs used for pain of cancer

Trade Name	Generic Name
Demerol	Meperidine
Dilaudid	Hydromorphone
Dolophine	Methadone
Lorcet, Lortab, Vicodin	Hydrocodone
Percocet, Percodan, Roxicet, Tylox	Oxycodone
Talwin	Pentazocine
Tylenol #3, Phenaphen #3, other	Codeine

For example, medications can be given in the traditional ways: orally or by injection into a muscle. Today there are many other effective ways to take narcotic medications for pain control. These include patches that allow the medication to be absorbed into the skin, or medications that can be absorbed easily when placed under the tongue. Other ways to deliver the narcotic for pain relief include a constant "drip" of medication through a needle placed in the fatty tissue just under the skin. Alternatively, a constant drip of narcotic through a needle placed in a vein is also effective. This allows the patient to control the rate of the pain medication and is commonly used as a postsurgical delivery system. Finally, injections and more constant "drips" can also be given around the nerves of the spinal cord for effective pain control.

Nerve Blocks

Another way effectively to stop pain is by injecting a chemical that permanently damages the nerve supplying the painful area so that it no longer produces pain. The injection may give prolonged and effective pain relief.

Surgically cutting the nerve(s) that supply the painful area can be an effective way to relieve cancer pain, but there may be other unwanted permanent effects on the other organs supplied by these nerves. This depends greatly on the individual situation. Be aware of this and discuss it with your physician.

Besides medications and injections, in recent years other methods of treating cancer pain have come into use. They continue to be used because in many patients they work to control pain. They also have the benefit of lowering the need for narcotics. These are discussed in chapter 5.

NERVE PAIN

When the diagnosis of nerve pain (neuropathy) is made, it helps to be sure that no additional causes of pain are present. For example, if there is also pain caused by arthritis, then it will be helpful to treat the arthritis. The most common types of nerve pain are those due to damage or irritation to the nerve endings, for example, the nerve pain after shingles infection. Nerve pain can happen in many areas of the body, including the feet and lower legs, a condition referred to as *peripheral neuropathy.*

Nerve Pain after Shingles

Treatment of the pain after shingles infection (discussed on p. 60) can be frustrating. Treatment with a medication directed against the virus itself is given with acyclovir (Zovirax) as early as possible, and continued for one week. Pain caused by shingles is treated with medications of the antidepressant type (see p. 76) which are usually added early. Other medications such as anticonvulsants can also be used for pain. Creams and rubs might be useful as well. Be very careful when using any cream or rub for nerve pain if a rash is present, since the skin surface can become more irritated.

Peripheral Neuropathy

When the diagnosis of peripheral neuropathy is made, an attempt to treat the underlying problem is first on the agenda. For example, diabetes mellitus is the most common cause of this type of nerve pain. Control of the blood glucose, which may be abnormally high in diabetes, can be an effective way of improving the nerve pain. It may take months to achieve, but it is well worth the effort.

Other causes of this peripheral neuropathy can be heavy alcohol use, poor nutrition, some medications, and blockage of arteries to the legs (usually due to atherosclerosis with as hardening and narrowing of the arteries). There are many other diseases such as cancer that can cause this problem. Each of these causes should be assessed and proper treatment begun. Unfortunately, in many cases, no specific underlying cause is found.

If the pain and abnormal sensitivity of the neuropathy continues, pain medications available over the counter may be enough. These include acetaminophen, ibuprofen, or aspirin in low doses taken only as needed.

If relief does not occur, narcotic pain medications are available. But since these often do not give good relief and their effects may be long-lasting, it is better that these be avoided to escape the risk of dependence.

Another group of medications used in chronic back pain are also often very effective in nerve pain. This is the group of anti-depressant-type medications (listed in table 3.5). These may give good to excellent pain relief. Because the doses of medication are usually low, the side effects are also low. These drug therapies are especially good in the relief of nerve pain in peripheral neuropathy. Other medications used include the anticonvulsants listed on p. 76 and can be tried if the above are not effective. These require monitoring by your doctor.

Some other methods that have been used with success in pain relief for peripheral neuropathy include Transcutaneous Electrical Nerve Stimulation (TENS) as discussed on p. 80. Some rubs and creams may give temporary relief as well. Capsaicin (Zostrix) is sometimes prescribed for use four times daily: this cream and others may give partial pain relief. If you have any questions, check with your doctor before using a cream or rub.

Finding a successful treatment for the pain of peripheral neuropathy can be frustrating for those with chronic nerve pain. Try to be patient as you go through the available medications and other treatments.

CARPAL TUNNEL SYNDROME

Carpal tunnel syndrome is a condition of pain and numbness caused by pressure on a nerve that supplies the hand. Treatment for carpal tunnel syndrome consists first of treating any underlying problem creating pressure on the nerve at the wrist. At times a simple splint for the wrist can be worn to help reduce swelling and pressure. A local injection at the wrist with a cortisone derivative may also reduce the swelling and relieve the pain and numbness. In some cases, surgery performed on an outpatient basis can permanently relieve the problem. Your doctor can tell you the best treatment for your own situation.

4

Get Moving to Reduce Your Pain

As stated in chapter 3, exercise and movement are vital to treatment programs for chronic pain. Let's look at the specific exercises recommended for use as part of your treatment. This chapter contains all the exercises, but you may need to select certain specific ones for your particular situation.

For example, for chronic neck pain due to arthritis, it is usually helpful to include strengthening and flexibility exercises for the neck, back and shoulders, since these give support to the neck. The stronger and more flexible these muscles, the better the support for the neck and the more likely it is that pain relief will occur.

For lower back pain, all the back exercises we have listed could be helpful. If you have questions about which exercises are best for your type of pain, check in chapter 3 for specific suggestions. *We strongly recommend that you always check with your doctor or physical therapist before you begin any exercises.*

RELIEF IS *NOT* IMMEDIATE

It is important to remember that several weeks to a few months must usually pass before an exercise program shows results. You may notice results earlier, but then again you may not. Be patient. The most effective program for good results will be to maintain the recommended number of repetitions for each exercise over a period of weeks.

GETTING STARTED WITH YOUR PROGRAM

As you begin the exercise program, remember to start *slowly*. Try one or two repetitions of an exercise twice daily, and slowly increase the number of repetitions as directed. If there is more pain when you finish, you may need to start again at only one or two repetitions. It is not necessary to increase repetitions dramatically to the full number: slow and steady increases are better. But make yourself do the exercises every day without fail as directed—*even* on your bad days.

If you don't understand an exercise or if it causes severe pain, stop and check with your doctor or physical therapist before continuing. If you have dizziness or shortness of breath with an exercise, then you should always stop until you talk with your doctor.

CONTINUE TO USE MOIST HEAT

Moist heat such as a warm shower or bath or a hot towel just before and during the exercises can greatly help your flexibility and may even make the exercises easier. As discussed on p. 67, a stool or chair with rubber tips for safety can be placed in the shower. If you use a shower, place a rubber mat in the tub and proceed cautiously so that you don't trip and fall. A warm swimming pool may be the best place of all to do these exercises, but a warm shower will also make them easier.

BACK EXERCISES

Buttock Raise

This exercise can be done while sitting, standing, or lying down. It strengthens the support for the back, pelvis, and legs.

Press the buttocks together and hold for six seconds. This will make you rise up slightly as shown in figure 4.1. Repeat, then gradually increase to five, then ten, then twenty repetitions, twice daily.

Pelvic Tilt

This strengthens the muscles of the back and abdomen. It can be done lying flat on your back either on the floor or in bed.

Put your arms over your head and keep your knees bent. Tighten

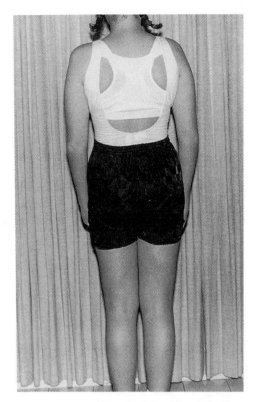

Figure 4.1

the muscles of the lower abdomen *and* your buttocks at the same time as shown in figure 4.2. This should flatten the back against the floor. Hold for six seconds, then repeat. Gradually increase up to five, then ten, then twenty repetitions, twice daily. If this is difficult to understand, talk to your physical therapist or doctor.

Bridging

This exercise strengthens the back muscles.

Lying on your back on the floor or in bed, bend your knees and lift your buttocks off the floor about four inches. Then tighten the buttocks and hip muscles to hold this position as shown in figure 4.3. Hold for six seconds. Then relax and lower the buttocks to the floor. Repeat, gradually increasing to five, then ten, then twenty of each exercise, twice daily.

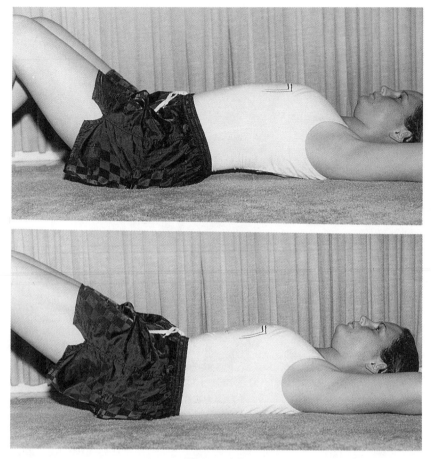

Figure 4.2

Partial Sit-Up

This exercise strengthens the back and abdominal muscles. You lie on the floor or bed to do this.

Lie on your back with your knees bent. Lift your head and shoulders off the floor as shown in figure 4.4 and hold this position for six seconds. Relax again flat on your back. Gradually increase from one to two to five, then ten exercises, twice daily, with the goal of eventually doing twenty of each exercise, twice daily. If you experience severe pain or shortness of breath, stop and talk to your doctor before you continue.

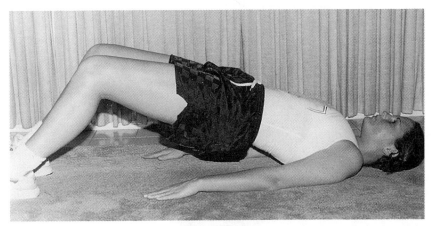

Figure 4.3

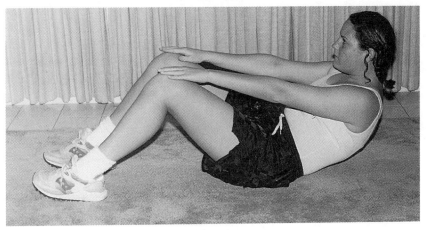

Figure 4.4

Back Extension

Lie on your stomach on the floor or bed. Raise your head, arms, and legs off the floor a few inches (see figure 4.5). Hold for six seconds. Repeat then gradually increase to five, then ten, then twenty of each exercise, twice daily. If you have severe pain, stop and talk to your doctor.

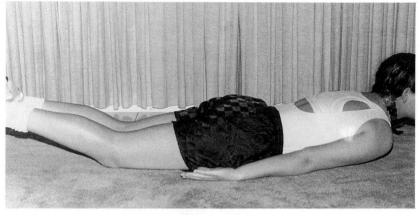

Figure 4.5

Cat-Camel Exercise

Start from a crawling position as shown in figure 4.6, with your hands directly below your shoulders. Then lower your head and arch your back (like a cat). Hold for six seconds and gradually raise your head and rest the back.

Increase this from one to two, then up to five, then ten repetitions, twice daily.

Spread Eagle

Stand spread eagle against a wall, with your hands on the wall. Arch your back slowly inward toward the wall as shown in figure 4.7. Gradually increase up to five, then ten repetitions, and repeat this exercise, twice daily.

Press-Ups

Lie on your stomach and push up with both arms while leaving hips down as shown in figure 4.8. The effort should come from the arms, and the back should remain relaxed. Start with a single repetition on the first day. Then as you are able, slowly increase the number to two, then three, and gradually increase until you can do ten repetitions each day. This may take weeks to achieve. Eventually, the goal is to be able to increase to twenty repetitions daily.

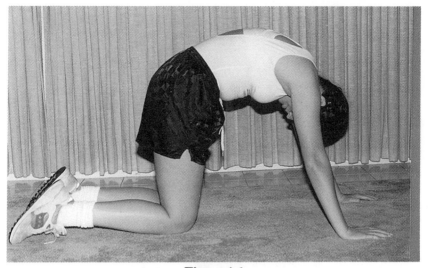

Figure 4.6

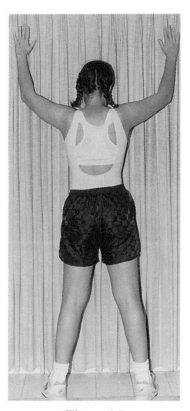

Figure 4.7

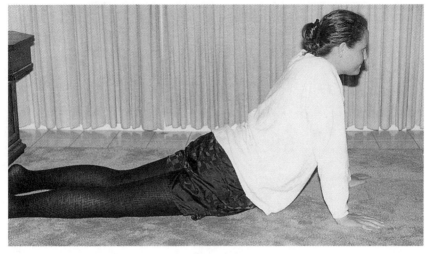

Figure 4.8

BACK-STRENGTHENING EXERCISES

One Leg Lift

Tighten the stomach muscles and lift your left leg straight out, keeping your back flat (do not arch your back), as shown in figure 4.9. Then do the same using the right leg. Gradually increase to three, then five, then ten, and finally twenty repetitions of each daily. If this seems too easy, then progress to the leg and arm lift.

Leg and Arm Lift

Tighten your stomach muscles and lift your left arm and right leg straight out, keeping your back flat. Then do the same using the right arm and left leg, as shown in figure 4.10. Gradually increase to three, then five, then ten, up to twenty repetitions of each daily.

Back Stretching

Lie on your back with your knees bent and feet flat on the floor or bed. Raise up your hands, move the arms to the right and the knees and legs to the left, as shown in figure 4.11. Then raise your hands, move your arms to the left and your knees to the right. Repeat and

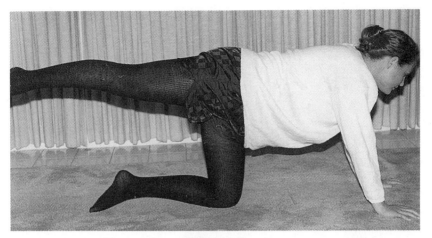

Figure 4.9

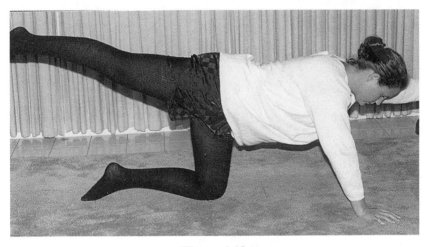

Figure 4.10

gradually increase to two, then five, then ten of each exercise, twice daily.

Bicycle

Lie on your back on the floor or bed and move your feet and legs as you pretend you are riding a bicycle (see figure 4.12). Do this for about ten seconds and gradually increase up to five and then ten or more repetitions, twice daily.

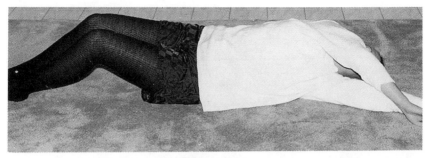

Figure 4.11

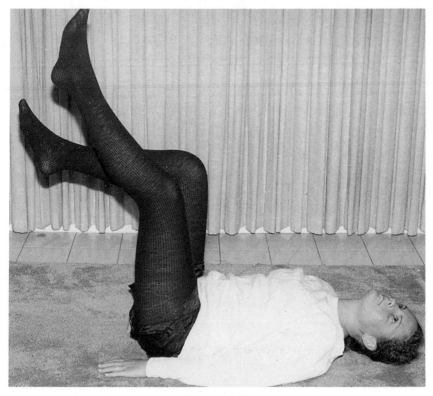

Figure 4.12

EXERCISES FOR NECK FLEXIBILITY

For each of these exercises, try one or two repetitions twice daily and gradually increase up to ten repetitions twice daily. If you have more pain or experience dizziness, then stop until you talk to your doctor.

Neck Flexion

This can be done either standing or sitting. Move the chin down to the chest as far as possible, as shown in figure 4.13. Go as far as you can with comfort. If pain persists with this exercise, then stop and see your doctor before continuing.

Neck Extension

Look up, bending the neck back as far as possible, as shown in figure 4.14. If you have dizziness or severe pain, then stop until you talk to your doctor or physical therapist.

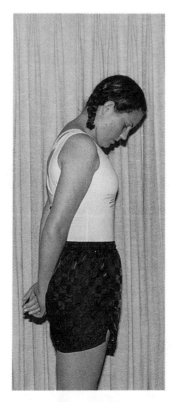

Figure 4.13

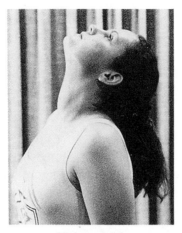

Figure 4.14

Lateral Bending

Move your left ear to the left shoulder, hold for five seconds, then return to the upright position. Then move your right ear to the right shoulder (see figure 4.15). Repeat.

Rotation

Turn as if you were looking over your right shoulder. You can go as far as possible if there is no pain. Then try looking over the left shoulder in the same manner (see figure 4.16).

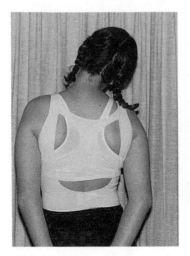

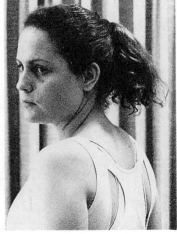

Figure 4.15   **Figure 4.16**

NECK ISOMETRIC EXERCISES

These are more advanced exercises to strengthen your neck muscles. You can try these after you feel comfortable with the other exercises, and the range of motion of the neck has improved as much as possible. If any of these exercises cause severe pain, stop until you talk to your doctor. Try beginning with one repetition then gradually increase up to five repetitions, twice daily, if there is no pain.

Flexion

This can be done either sitting or standing (see figure 4.17). With your hand on your forehead, push the head against your hand while your hand resists the movement. Hold and count to six.

Extension

Put your hands on the back of your head and push backward against your hand with your head, while you resist the movement with your hands (see figure 4.18). Hold for six seconds.

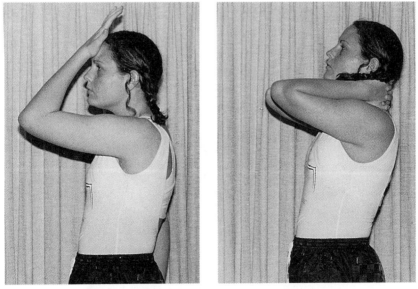

Figure 4.17   **Figure 4.18**

Lateral Bending

Put the palm of your left hand on the side of your head above your ear. Now try to move your head against your hand, but push back with your hand. Hold for six seconds. Then repeat the exercise using your right hand on the right side of your head above your ear (see figure 4.19), holding again for six seconds.

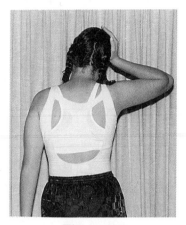

Figure 4.19

Rotation

Put your left hand on the side of your head near your left forehead. Then try to look over your left shoulder while you push against the movement with your left hand (see figure 4.20). Hold this for six seconds.

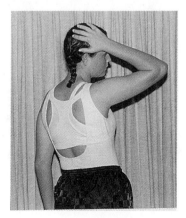

Figure 4.20

Dorsal Glide

The purpose of this exercise is to improve the forward head posture.

Sit in a chair and tuck your chin in (see figure 4.21). Slide your head and neck back over your shoulders, keeping your head tucked in all the while. Hold for five seconds and gradually increase from one up to five repetitions daily.

Thoracic Extensions

Sit in a chair that will support your back. Tighten your stomach muscles to prevent your lower back from arching. Bend your upper back backward, as shown in figure 4.22. Hold for five seconds and gradually increase from one up to five repetitions daily.

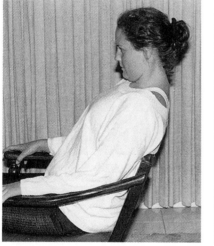
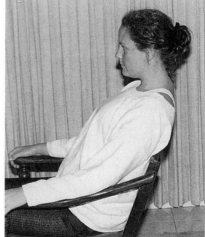

Figure 4.21   **Figure 4.22**

SHOULDER EXERCISES

These exercises can increase the strength and flexibility of the shoulders. Start with one of each exercise, then increase to two, then gradually increase to five, then ten, and on up to twenty of each exercise, twice daily. If there is any unusual pain, stop the exercise and talk with your doctor immediately.

External Rotation

Sit or stand with your hands clasped behind your head as in figure
4.23. Then try to touch your elbows in front of your chin, moving
your elbows out to the sides as much as possible in the process.

Internal Rotation

While sitting or standing, place your hands crossed behind your back;
then try to raise them up higher on the back (see figure 4.24).

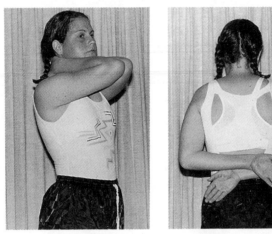

Figure 4.23   **Figure 4.24**

Flexion

While standing or sitting, raise your arms straight overhead, as shown
in figure 4.25.

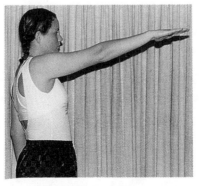

Figure 4.25

Abduction

In this exercise, while sitting or standing, raise your arms straight out to your side and up over your head (see figure 4.26a).

Then raise your arms out to your sides (see figure 4.26b), first the left arm, then the right, and make big circles.

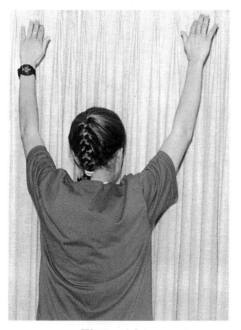

Figure 4.26a

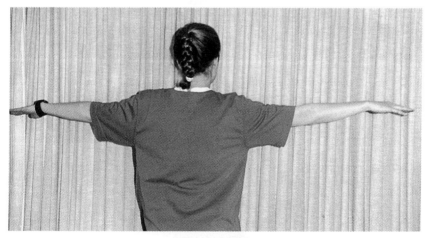

Figure 4.26b

Rotation

While sitting or standing, roll your shoulders in a forward circle (begin with shoulder shrugging movement). Then reverse and move the shoulders back in the opposite direction, as shown in figure 4.27.

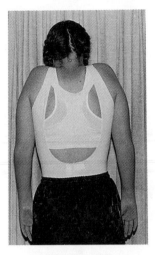

Figure 4.27

HIP EXERCISES

Flexion

These exercises are actually good not only for the hips but for the back and the knees. You can do these exercises on the floor or in bed.

Bend your left knee to the chest, then bend your right knee to the chest. If needed, you can help by using your hands to help bend your knee (see figure 4.28a). Repeat, alternating left and right knees. Try to increase to five, then ten, then up to twenty repetitions, twice daily.

Pull both knees to the chest at the same time as in figure 4.28b. Hold this position for six seconds and then slowly rock from side to side while holding your knees. Gently let your legs down. Repeat, gradually increasing to five, then ten, then twenty repetitions, twice daily.

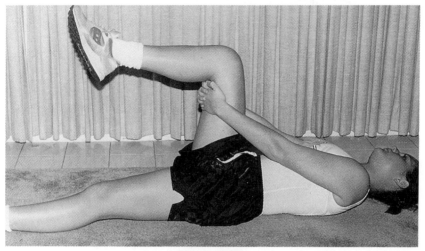

Figure 4.28a

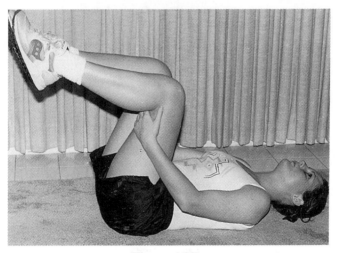

Figure 4.28b

Abduction

This can be done lying on the floor or in bed. While lying on your back (with your knees straight or slightly bent), slide your left leg out to the side, then return to the starting position (see figure 4.29). Now do the same movement with your right leg. Gradually increase up to five, then ten, then twenty repetitions for each leg, twice daily.

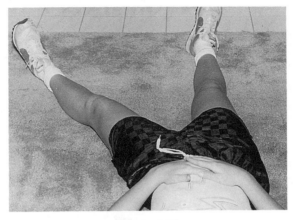

Figure 4.29

Extension

This can be done lying on your stomach on the floor or in bed. Keep your knee straight and lift your left thigh straight up off the floor (or bed) about eight inches (see figure 4.30). Hold this position while you count to six. Repeat with the right leg, then alternate legs and gradually increase up to five, then ten, then twenty repetitions, twice daily. If there is severe pain, stop until you talk to your doctor.

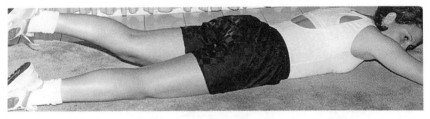

Figure 4.30

Rotation

Lie on your back on the floor or in bed. With your knees straight, turn your knees in and touch the toes of your feet foot together (see figure 4.31a). Now turn the knees out (see figure 4.31b). Repeat this, gradually increasing up to five, then ten, then twenty repetitions, twice daily.

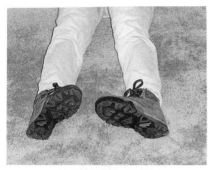 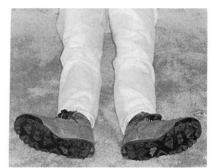

Figure 4.31a   **Figure 4.31b**

KNEE AND LEG EXERCISES

Extension

This exercise can strengthen the muscles of the thighs (quadriceps muscles), which offer a major support for the knee. You can do this while reading, watching television, or riding in an airplane. The more you do it, the stronger the support will be for your knees.

While sitting in a chair, support your leg on a chair or table and straighten your knee as much as possible (see figure 4.32). Then tighten your knee cap (push the knee down) until you feel the muscles of your thigh tighten. Keep that muscle tight and count to six. Relax, and then repeat, gradually increasing up to five, then ten, then fifteen repetitions, twice daily.

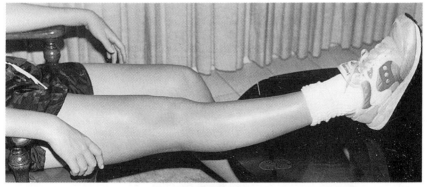

Figure 4.32

Straight Leg Raise

While lying on the floor or in bed, bend your knee slightly as shown, or bend one knee to the chest if you have chronic back pain. Raise the other leg slowly while keeping the back firmly on the floor or bed (see figure 4.33). Raise your leg as high as you can, but stop if your back begins to arch. Hold and count to six. Lower your leg, then repeat the stops for the opposite leg. Repeat for both legs, gradually increasing to five, then ten, then twenty repetitions, twice daily. If you have severe pain with this exercise, stop immediately and talk to your doctor.

Flexion

You can do this on the floor or in bed. Lie on your stomach and bend your knees as far as you can toward your back (see figure 4.34). Straighten your knee, then repeat, gradually increasing up to five, then ten, then twenty repetitions, twice daily.

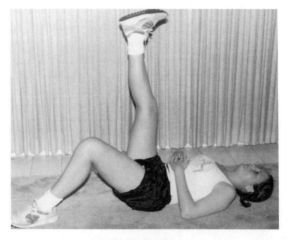

Figure 4.33

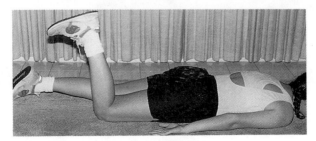

Figure 4.34

POSTURE EXERCISES

Posture exercises strengthen the muscles that help maintain good body alignment. This will help increase flexibility and make daily activities easier. If you are bothered by back pain, improving posture will result in less pressure on the spine and can lessen pain. It can help you achieve your goals in chronic pain—increased activity with improved pain control.

Deep Breathing

Lying on the floor or in bed with your hands behind your head and knees bent, breathe deeply and raise your chest while filling your lungs completely as shown in figure 4.35. Hold for a few seconds. Then exhale as you draw in your abdomen. Gradually increase up to five, then ten repetitions, twice daily.

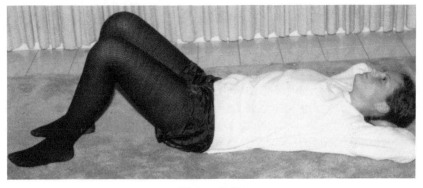

Figure 4.35

Arms Back

While standing, lift your elbows to shoulder level and straighten the arms backward (see figure 4.36). Hold for six seconds. Repeat, then gradually increase up to five, then ten, then twenty repetitions, twice daily.

Swinging Arms

Standing and relaxed, with arms crossed in front, swing your hands up, outward and over your head while reaching backward, as shown in figure 4.37. Then lower your arms. Repeat, then gradually increase to five, then ten, then twenty repetitions, twice daily.

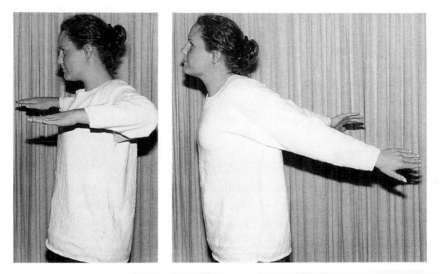

Figure 4.36   **Figure 4.37**

Swinging Arms Diagonally

Standing relaxed with both hands down to one side, move your hands diagonally across the front of your body, then up and over your head (see figure 4.38). Try to inhale on the upswing. Then gradually lower the hands and arms as you exhale on the downswing. Repeat but start on the opposite side and reverse the direction of the upswing. Repeat both directions and gradually increase up to five, then ten repetitions, twice daily.

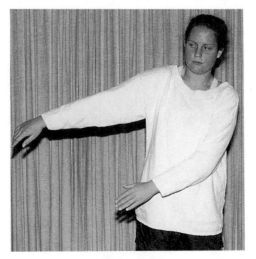

Figure 4.38

STRENGTHENING EXERCISES

Once you can do twenty of each exercise twice daily and maintain a regular program for a few weeks, you will begin to notice improvement in flexibility and strength. You can increase the exercises to build stronger muscles in more than one way.

Isometric exercises use resistance to allow increase in muscle strength without movement of the joints. For example, the exercise in figure 4.39 is an isometric exercise for the neck. The strength of the resistance should be low at first and very gradually increased as you feel comfortable.

Elastic bands, available through any physical therapist, can be used in isometric exercises, as shown in figure 4.40. These come in different levels of resistance from light to heavy. Start with the lightest level and gradually increase, if you can do so comfortably.

Weights can be used. Choose light weights of one to two pounds. These can be added to the hands or feet as your usual exercises are done to help build muscle strength. Weights with Velcro straps, which can be strapped to the wrist or ankle, are available at sporting goods stores.

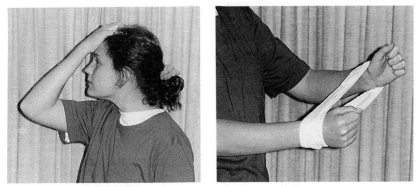

Figure 4.39   **Figure 4.40**

Shoulder Isometric Exercises

Using an elastic or rubber band obtained from your physical therapist, pull both arms apart as shown in figure 4.41. The band should be placed just above the wrists. When the band is tight, pull one arm upward and one downward, and hold for six seconds. Then pull the other arm upward and the opposite downward, and hold for six seconds. The time spent holding can be slowly increased from six seconds as you feel comfortable, if there is no pain.

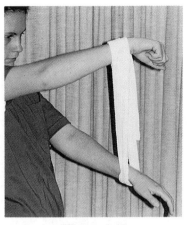

Figure 4.41

Elbow Isometric Exercises

Place the bands just above your wrists. With the elbows bent, pull one elbow toward you and straighten out the other elbow, as shown in figure 4.42. When the band is tight, hold for six seconds. Repeat in the opposite direction. The time spent holding can be increased, if there is no pain.

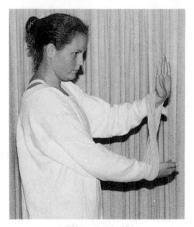

Figure 4.42

Hip Isometric Exercises

While sitting in a chair put your hands on the outer part of your upper legs. Then push your upper legs inward with your hands while you try to push your legs outward (see figure 4.43a).

Now with your hands on the inside part of your thighs, try to push your thighs inward while you push them outward with your hands (see figure 4.43b).

Repeat each of these, then gradually increase up to five, then ten, then twenty repetitions, twice daily.

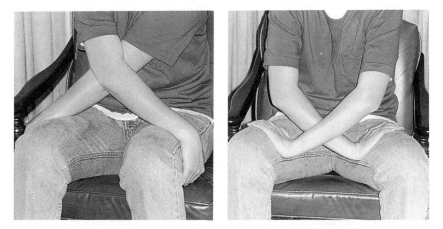

| Figure 4.43a | Figure 4.43b |

Exercises with Weights

With one- or two-pound weights strapped on your wrists, raise your right arm upward toward your head and back to your side, as shown in figure 4.44a. Repeat with the other arm, then gradually increase up to five, then ten times daily with both arms.

Try making a circle with your arm outstretched and your elbow straight, and as you do so, gradually increase the size of the circle. Repeat, then gradually increase the repetitions to five, then ten times, twice daily.

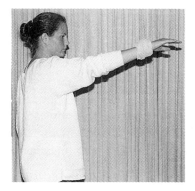

Figure 4.44a

With the weight now strapped to your ankle and while lying on your back on the floor or in bed, slide one leg out to your side, then back to the middle. Repeat with the opposite leg, then gradually increase up to five, then ten repetitions, twice daily for both legs.

Try sitting in a chair with the weights strapped on your ankles. Then straighten your right knee, hold for a few seconds, and then lower your foot back to the floor (see figure 4.44b). Repeat with the opposite knee, then gradually repeat up to five, then ten times, twice daily.

These exercises improve neck support by increasing the flexibility and strength of the muscles of the neck. These can be done either standing or sitting. Use the range of motion exercises to get the maximum movement. Then you can try some isometric strengthening exercises.

When you use resistance to help build strength in the muscles, start with least resistance and increase very gradually. It may be a good idea to have the help of a physical therapist for some exercises.

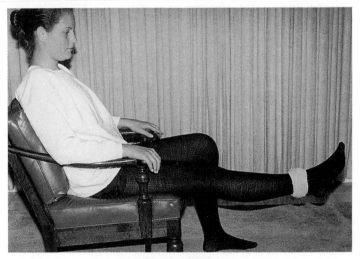

Figure 4.44b

ELBOW AND ARM EXERCISES

Flexion and Extension

Sitting or standing, bend your right elbow and bring your hand to touch your right shoulder, then straighten your arm out completely (see figure 4.45). Repeat this with both arms, increasing up to twenty repetitions for each arm twice daily.

Pronation and Supination

Turn the palm of your hand up and then down. Repeat and gradually increase up to twenty repetitions twice daily (see figure 4.46).

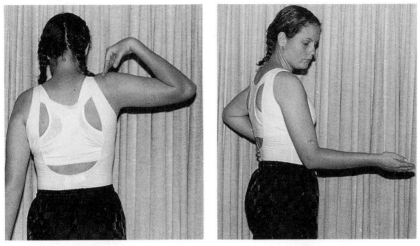

Figure 4.45   **Figure 4.46**

WRIST, HAND, AND FINGER EXERCISES

Flexion and Extension for Wrists

With your arm on a table, counter, or chair, extend one hand down over the edge of the table or chair. Use the other hand to bend the hand at the wrist up then down as far as possible without pain (see figure 4.47a). Repeat, increasing up to twenty repetitions twice daily.

Now, placing your hand flat on a table, move the hand at the wrist so that your entire hand moves to the right, then to the left, as far as possible, as shown in figure 4.47b. You can use the other hand for assistance if needed. Repeat, increasing up to twenty repetitions daily.

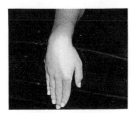   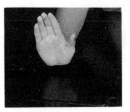

Figure 4.47a   **Figure 4.47b**

Finger Flexion and Extension

Close the fingers, making a fist (see figure 4.48a), then open and extend the fingers as straight as possible. Repeat this, gradually increasing up to twenty of each exercise twice daily. You can use a foam or a sponge ball about the size of a tennis ball (available at any toy store) to squeeze the fingers together (see figure 4.48b). Release and extend the fingers.

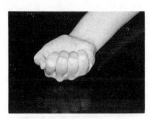
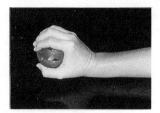

Figure 4.48a   **Figure 4.48b**

Finger Curls

If your fingers are stiff, try to curl each finger down and bend each joint in the fingers as much as possible, as in figure 4.49. Don't force the movement, but you can use one hand to help curl the fingers of the other. Repeat and gradually increase up to twenty times for each finger, twice daily.

Finger Extension

Straighten each finger as you press your palm flat on the table, as shown in figure 4.50. Don't force this movement if there is severe pain. This can be done twice daily.

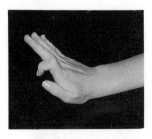
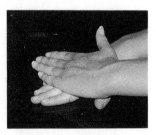

Figure 4.49   **Figure 4.50**

Thumb and Finger

For grasp and pinch, try to form the letter O with your thumb and each one of your fingers separately (see figure 4.51). Make a good round O, then straighten the finger and move to the next finger. Repeat for each finger, gradually increasing up to twenty repetitions twice daily.

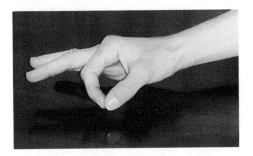

Figure 4.51

Finger Spreading

Spread your fingers wide apart, then close them together as tightly as you can, as shown in figures 4.52a and 4.52b. Do this twice daily, increasing up to twenty repetitions each session.

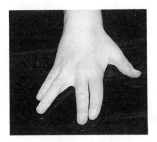

Figure 4.52a

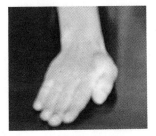

Figure 4.52b

ANKLE AND FOOT EXERCISES

These exercises are easy to do and can be performed while seated almost anywhere. Raise your toes as high as you can with your heels on the floor (see figure 4.53a). Then press your toes to the floor and raise the heels as high as you can (see figure 4.53b). Finally, rotate the ankles in a circle. Repeat each exercise, gradually increasing to five, then ten, then twenty of each one, twice daily.

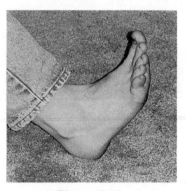

Figure 4.53a

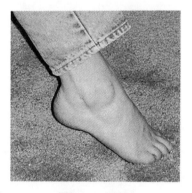

Figure 4.53b

5

Other Treatments for Pain

OTHER INJECTIONS FOR PAIN

When other treatment is not enough, there are several types of injections other than trigger point injections available for chronic pain. These are injections around the spine in specific areas using a local anesthetic and a cortisone derivative which may give pain relief that lasts for weeks or even months. If the result is excellent the injections may be repeated. Sometimes a temporary interruption of the pain may produce a longer-lasting effect, perhaps by interrupting the constant pain. These nerve blocks are discussed on pp. 81–82 and 104–105.

LONGER-TERM NARCOTIC INJECTIONS

There are many other treatment methods available for chronic pain if the basic treatment program brings little or no relief. A catheter can be surgically inserted for longer-term use of such drugs as narcotics for pain control. This method is used mainly in the treatment of cancer patients, and it is effective, but it can also be quite expensive. A device called a port is installed, usually on the chest, which is used to inject medication as often as needed. This can also be done to allow a continuous pump of medication for pain control. The pump can be made to allow medication (such as morphine) to be delivered to the blood through a vein or around the spinal cord. This device causes little or no restriction of movement. Lower doses of medications are needed for pain relief when given in this way since it is a much more direct route to the source of pain. A trial of this treatment on a temporary basis is done before long-term treatment commences. Many different types of pain, such as cancer pain or severe, debilitating back pain, may respond to this treatment.

NERVE STIMULATION AND PERMANENT NERVE BLOCK

Just as Transcutaneous Electrical Nerve Stimulation (TENS) is used to control nerve pain, a longer-lasting type of electrical stimulation of the spinal nerves is possible. An electrode is placed near certain portions of the spinal column to affect the area of chronic pain. A battery (which can also be implanted) is used to supply small electrical stimulations that attempt to control pain by blocking the pathways of the pain messages from nerves.

The idea is that the electrical signal produced blocks the "pain message" before it goes to the brain. Before an electrode is planted, a test trial of a temporary electrode must be successful in reducing pain. Many pain problems, such as back or cancer pain, can be treated in this way.

Permanent blockage of the nerve may be accomplished by injecting a damaging drug or by other equally invasive methods. However, these treatments should be undertaken only after a complete consultation with your doctor. Often damage to other parts of the treated nerve occurs as well. If the nerve supply to muscles or other organs is permanently blocked, then such unwanted effects as muscle weakness could well be permanent. If this method is used, it should be carefully planned to give maximum benefit without any unnecessary or unwanted side effects.

Surgery can be used to permanently damage the nerve supply in an effort to control the pain. Unfortunately, there is no assurance that the pain won't eventually return, this time with heightened severity. Since this procedure cannot be reversed, careful planning is needed. Damaging the afflicted nerve is a treatment that is reserved for only a few patients who have not responded favorably to any other pain control treatments.

ACUPUNCTURE

In acupuncture, fine needles are placed at specific points along the body in lines called meridians. The exact way in which acupuncture acts is unknown, but it may act through the nervous system or by release of endorphins, the body's natural pain-relieving chemicals. The procedure involves the needles being in place for fifteen to thirty minutes, with or without twisting the needles or attaching a small electrical current. Eight to ten treatments may be needed to judge whether relief will occur.

Acupuncture has been practiced in Chinese medicine for centuries.

Some patients find relief that is worthwhile, but the response for each person cannot be predicted. Acupuncture is fairly simple and inexpensive, and may have a place for those patients for whom nothing else has been helpful. Just as with other pain treatments, acupuncture can be continued if it gives you relief.

RELAXATION RESPONSE

There are many factors that allow us to experience pain. Researchers have found that a person's emotional and mental states are important. It is believed that positive thoughts, feeling relaxed, and a general sense of well-being can lower the overall pain; negative thoughts, anxiety, and worry may allow much more pain.

Achieving relaxation through the relaxation response can help a person reduce some of the emotional stress of pain. This is done by developing an inner quiet and peacefulness, a calming of negative thoughts and worries, and a mental focus away from the pain itself.

Relaxation response is a particular response of the body which can be very helpful in chronic pain. The experience of pain, expecially chronic pain, is a major source of stress, both physically and mentally. The use of the relaxation response came from research which showed that this can reduce stress, anxiety, tension, and actually reduce pain.

The physical stress of pain comes from the hurting itself and the body's response to the pain. For example, a common response of the body to the stress of pain is for muscles to become tense and tight. Tightened muscles can cause pain which may actually increase the amount of pain we feel. A vicious cycle of ever-increasing levels of pain begins. Effective relaxation may offer the benefits of reducing excess muscle tension, thereby eliminating the "added pain" that stiffened muscles cause.

The stress of being in chronic pain also puts important mental and emotional demands on a person. Chronic pain affects one's mood and causes irritability, impatience, and higher levels of frustration. As will be discussed in chapter 7, depression commonly occurs as well.

It is natural for those with chronic pain to become preoccupied with the hurting and find it difficult, if not impossible, to think about anything else. Also, the pain may put a heavy emotional demand on sufferers through worry and apprehension about the pain getting worse.

While pain is regarded by many people as mainly physical, it is also known that emotional factors can play an important role in the overall pain experience. For example, think of the people who cut a finger but do not have pain until they look at their finger and see the blood!

Relaxation—which can be learned even by people experiencing severe chronic pain—can offer a real potential to reduce physical strain and negative thoughts—and increase people's ability to self-manage their pain.

Achieving relaxation uses a mental approach to activity in general rather than any one specific activity. For each of us, many different activities or routines may be relaxing, depending on our particular mental attitude. And what may be relaxing for one person can be frustrating or tension-producing for another. For example, some of us may find it calming and soothing to lie quietly and listen to a certain type of music; others may gain more relaxation from reading an enjoyable book. Remember that true relaxation involves more than just being still or physical inactivity. You may not be relaxed just sitting in front of the TV. Some even have a high level of tension in their bodies and minds during sleep. An example would be those who toss and turn at night or who grind their teeth while asleep.

Relaxation is a skill that all people have the potential to develop. Some of us are naturally better at relaxing than others, but we can all learn to relax effectively. Much like learning to play the piano or tennis, becoming good at relaxation involves time, patience, and practice. Learning to relax deeply and effectively is a skill that develops gradually and cannot be rushed or hurried.

To begin your own relaxation program, you might try following these steps. During some part of your day, set aside a period of about twenty minutes that you can devote to relaxation practice. This can be in the morning, afternoon, or evening; just pick a time when you may have few obligations or commitments so you won't feel hurried or rushed.

As much as possible, remove outside distractions that can disrupt your concentration: turn off the radio, the TV, even the ringer on the telephone if need be. During practice, it is important either to lie flat or recline comfortably so that your whole body is supported, relieving as much tension or tightness in your muscles as possible. This is hard to do upright, since your muscles must be tightened to maintain the position. You can use a pillow or cushion under your head if this helps.

During the twenty-minute period, remain as still as possible; try to direct your thoughts away from events of the day. Try to focus your thoughts as much as possible on the immediate moment, and eliminate any outside thoughts which may compete for your attention. Focus entirely on yourself and the different kinds of feelings or sensations you may notice throughout your body. Notice which parts of your body feel relaxed and loose, and which parts feel tense.

As you go through these steps, in your own way try to imagine that every muscle in your body is now becoming loose, relaxed, and free of any excess tension. Picture all of the muscles in your body beginning to unwind; imagine them beginning to go loose and limp.

As you do this, concentrate on making your breating nice and even, breathing slowly and in a regular fashion. With each breath as you exhale, picture your muscles becoming even more relaxed, as if with each breath you can somehow breathe the tension away. At the end of twenty minutes, take a few moments to study and focus on the feelings and sensations you have been able to achieve. Notice whether areas that felt tight and tense at first now feel more loose and relaxed, and whether any areas of tension or tightness remain.

Don't be surprised if the relaxed feeling you achieve begins to fade and dissipate once you get up and return to your normal activities. Many people find that it is only after several weeks of daily, consistent practice that they are able to maintain the relaxed feeling beyond the practice session itself.

A variety of formal or structured approaches to relaxation training can be effective. One of these widely used techniques is progressive muscle relaxation, beginning with one area of the body and slowly moving to all areas. Other methods are controlled breathing exercises, the use of mental imagery, and meditation. If you find it hard to relax on your own or if you are interested in learning more about an individual approach for relaxation and pain management, then talk with your doctor. It might be a good idea to see a clinical psychologist who specializes in working with these problems. Whether you use the techniques we have discussed or choose formal training by a professional, learning to relax effectively can help control chronic pain, increase your activity, and lessen the impact of pain on your overall lifestyle.

MUSIC THERAPY

Some less common ways to treat pain include the use of music. Some researchers have found that in some cancer patients the use of various types of music can achieve better control of pain by patients. One study found that most patients had some response and almost half had at least a moderate response to pain with "music therapy." This cannot be the only treatment for chronic pain, but for many patients the partial relief offered by music therapy can be very welcome. The way in which music therapy relieves pain may be by helping the body's relaxation response, as discussed on p. 141.

BIOFEEDBACK

Biofeedback is similar in some ways to the relaxation response. In this method, a machine helps you to understand when you are relaxing your body and which emotions can help or hurt pain control. With this method taught by a qualified licensed psychologist, the patient can control responses of the body and better control pain. For example, in biofeedback training you are connected to a machine that shows when you are actually physically relaxing your body. This is measured by the tension in muscles, the amount of sweat, or by the temperature of the skin. The biofeedback instructor can use these readings to help you learn to control the responses of your body. Once this is accomplished, you can then control the body's responses at other times as well, including times of stress. This technique can be helpful in pain control.

COGNITIVE THERAPY

Another, newer way to help cancer pain is to change the beliefs, thoughts, and behaviors that affect how we perceive pain, and to learn specific ways of coping with the pain. This is called cognitive therapy. Pain sufferers learn to control their own beliefs and reactions to pain. This can help eliminate the feelings that make pain worse. For example, a person who felt helpless from chronic back pain and was constantly complaining used this method with improved pain control and increased ability to work.

Individual goals can be set, such as increasing specific activity or work levels. The person is taught newer ways to respond to the pain, which in turn develops better skill at dealing with pain. This does not eliminate the pain, of course, but may help make it tolerable. A psychologist who specializes in the treatment of pain can teach this method of pain control.

HYPNOSIS

Hypnosis has been tried successfully to help chronic pain. It should be used to help other methods of pain control (such as exercises and medications). All persons are not suitable for hypnosis, but a qualified therapist can tell if you would benefit. With hypnosis, the therapist will try to find ways that will allow you to control the pain process. Self-hypnosis is often used. The exact way in which hypnosis actually works is not known, but suggestions for control of feelings in one part of the body are taught. Then these feelings are transferred to control the painful part of the body. A true "hypnotic state" is not always necessary to be successful.

Hypnosis is not meant for everyone and may not work in every person. You should find a qualified clinical psychologist or psychiatrist to help you decide if hypnosis would be helpful and safe for you.

INDIVIDUAL PAIN RELIEF

The best results occur when the most effective combination of all available methods for each individual patient are found for pain relief. As always, everyone is different, and some forms of pain control will be valuable for certain patients and less useful for others. The team of patient and staff must work together to find the most effective combination of methods for pain relief. If adequate pain relief is still not found, then a good idea would be to consider a comprehensive cancer pain clinic. These clinics specialize in all the available ways to control pain in cancer patients. Results are good in these centers, with most patients finding relief.

SUPPORT GROUPS

Support groups are extremely helpful to people with chronic pain. In a support group, people suffering from similar problems can share their situations and receive comfort and encouragement from each other. The latest available treatments can be discussed and members can give coping suggestions while affirming the positive experiences of others. The assurance is given that "someone else knows what I am going through" as people share their struggle in living with chronic pain.

If no local support groups exist in your area, there are organizations that help you begin one. One such group is the American Chronic Pain Association, which was founded in 1980 to reach out to people with chronic pain and to offer a support system and group activities. To date, there are over 700 chapters in the United States, Canada, New Zealand, Australia, Mexico, and Russia. Members learn to use physician-approved stretching exercises, relaxation techniques, assertiveness training methods, sleep hygiene, nutrition, family involvement, and a better understanding of the feelings pain creates to live a fuller life. The American Chronic Pain Association also publishes a workbook and teaches coping skills.

The National Chronic Pain Outreach Association, Inc. (NCPOA), is a nonprofit organization that was also established in 1980. Its purpose is to lessen the suffering of people with chronic pain by educating pain sufferers, healthcare professionals, and the public about chronic pain and its management. The NCPOA publishes a quarterly magazine titled *Lifeline* and offers informational brochures.

Both organizations can give you information, names of support groups, and other resources. The American Chronic Pain Association's address is P.O. Box 850, Rocklin, CA 95677; its telephone number is (916) 632-0922. You may contact the National Chronic Pain Outreach Association, Inc., at 7979 Old Georgetown Rd., Suite 100E, Bethesda, MD 20814, or call (301) 652-4948.

For information on accredited chronic pain management programs in your area, contact the Commission on Accreditation of Rehabilitation Facilities, 101 North Wilmont Road, Suite 500, Tucson, AZ 85711, (800) 444-8991. The American Pain Society, a group of health providers, can give additional information about pain units in your area. Call them at (708) 966-5595.

Other toll free numbers for assistance and referrals for specific types of chronic pain include:

- Arthritis Foundation Information Line, (800) 283-7800; 9 A.M. to 7 P.M. weekdays except holidays.

- National Headache Foundation, (800) 843-2256; 10 A.M. to 6 P.M., weekdays except holidays.

- National Cancer Institute Cancer Information Service, (800) 4-CANCER; 9 A.M. to 4:30 P.M., all time zones, weekdays.

- National Mental Health Association, (800) 969-6642; 24 hours, every day (for brochures on stress, depression, and other mental health problems, and referral to counseling groups and professionals).

NONSTANDARD TREATMENT

For almost all of the chronic pain problems we have reviewed thus far, there are no easy cures. But there will always be many "wonderful" treatments offered by concerned friends and family members who honestly want to help you and would genuinely like to see you have pain relief.

Unfortunately, there will also be many "wonderful" treatments offered by some whose main motive is to profit from your pain. With no relief after months and years from standard medical treatment, it is understandable that these alternative treatments begin to look more and more attractive. It becomes very hard not to try at least some treatments. After all, they seem reasonable, and "someone" said they worked great! And you may feel a bit pressured not to offend the friend who offers it.

You may worry that if you try one of the nonstandard treatments, your physician will become angry. On the other hand, you don't want to miss any possible improvement in pain, even a small amount of relief.

Some treatments may be standard and acceptable but the information you are given is misleading. For example, an article in a newspaper discussed a treatment for pain that used an operation to place a permanent electrical stimulator in the spinal cord (see p. 140). This was seen by many chronic pain sufferers who had great interest in trying it. But the truth is that this treatment has many risks and limitations and is extremely expensive. It is really intended for only a few patients, those who have unsuccessfully tried all other treatments. But simply reading the article gave a much different impression.

The best advice is to talk with your doctor about each treatment as you discover it; but given the number of new and "wonderful" treatments that come out each year, this may be difficult to do. What if one or more of the treatments *could* help safely? How can you get the benefit of any good that can come from such "wonderful" treatments, but avoid the bad ones? How can you tell if the treatment is being needlessly avoided by your doctor?

It helps if you become your own *expert.* Learn about your problem from your doctor and ask for other sources of information. Become familiar with the available ways to treat the pain and the underlying problem. *The more you know, the better you can understand and participate in your own care.*

Most of the "wonderful" treatments that *should be avoided* have some characteristics in common: (1) they usually promise a quick and easy cure or relief, (2) there is usually a supplier waiting to sell you the treatment, (3) they have not been tested carefully as the U.S. government requires of new treatments, and (4) they may claim that doctors are covering up the treatment.

PROTECT YOURSELF

Some questions you should ask about any possible new treatment for chronic pain include the following:

- How old is the treatment?
- What side effects does it have?
- Has it been tested in trials approved by the U.S. government?
- Will the treatment still be around next year?
- Is it regulated by the U.S. government?
- What has happened to other similar treatments over the years?

If a "wonderful" treatment is harmless but won't delay proper medical diagnosis and treatment, then it is acceptable to try. For example, many creams, rubs, and ointments, if not taken internally, would be acceptable. Follow the directions carefully. If there is no irritation of the skin, and there is pain relief, then use it as directed. Most patients in our clinic have tried all sorts of lotions or rubs at some time. They often feel better just knowing that they haven't missed a potentially good remedy.

It is important to know when a substance may be dangerous to your health, and you should avoid any substance that must be taken internally (unless you have had it approved by your doctor). For example, rattlesnake meat is a common remedy in some areas for many illnesses, including arthritis and back pain. However, some types of capsules containing rattlesnake meat have been shown to cause diarrhea and severe illness.

If you have questions about a new treatment, talk to your doctor and make sure it is safe to use. This can allow you to take advantage of newer treatments but avoid those that may cause more harm than relief.

COMPREHENSIVE PAIN CLINICS

If after months of trying various of the above methods to reduce chronic pain there is still no improvement in pain control and little or no increase in activity, it would be wise to consider being evaluated in a comprehensive pain clinic. Many pain clinics may have one type of treatment that is emphasized over the others. The most common are medical treatment, nerve blocks, the use of physical therapy, and psychological approaches to pain control. Each area can offer improvement in pain and activity to those with chronic limitation brought on by pain (see figure 5.1).

Comprehensive pain clinics combine all standard methods for pain evaluation and control. This includes medical evaluation and physical therapy measures, as well as psychological evaluation and treatment. Many patients who have not responded to earlier treatments experience improvement in pain, increase their activity level, use less medication, and eventually return to work.

These clinics usually see the more severe cases of pain since, by the time clients, seek out the clinics they have tried most of the other treatments. Even with these more difficult problems, many comprehensive pain clinics can help: patients are up to twice as likely to return to work after therapy at a clinic than with other treatments alone. In fact, forty to sixty percent of the patients treated in many comprehensive clinics return to work.

Considering that these patients have not responded to most treatments, the figures are encouraging. These persons have less pain, improved activity, and use less healthcare. Remember, for example, that most of the cost of back pain—as much as $50 to $75 billion—is due to chronic back pain. Even a small amount of improvement in these cases can result in major savings in health costs as well as in suffering.

Consider a comprehensive pain clinic evaluation if all the other therapeutic measures have failed. And remember, the longer you remain out of work due to chronic pain, the more likely you are never to return to work. The earlier the treatment (once the necessary treatment is made clear), the better your chance of improvement so that you can return to work.

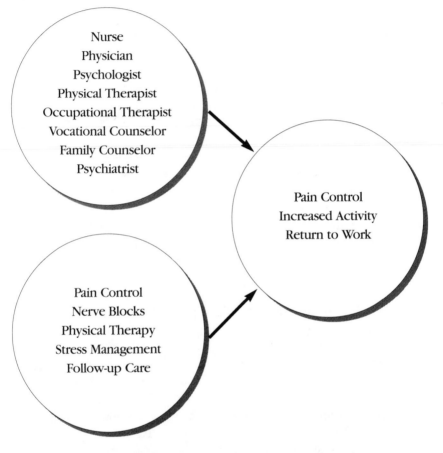

Figure 5.1. Diagram of a comprehensive pain clinic

GUIDELINES FOR SELECTING
A PAIN MANAGEMENT PROGRAM

A multidisciplinary pain program in a chronic pain clinic can provide the necessary skills, medical intervention, and direction to cope effectively with chronic pain. The following information* will help those in pain go about locating a pain management program in their immediate area, about what to look for in a well-defined pain program, and what other issues to consider.

1. *Make sure you locate a legitimate program:*
   - Facilities that offer pain management should include several specific components (listed below).

   - The Commission on Accreditation of Rehabilitation Facilities (CARF) (telephone: [800] 444-8991) can provide a listing of accredited pain programs in your area. (Your health insurance may require that the unit be CARF-accredited in order for you to receive reimbursement.) You can also contact the American Pain Society, a group of healthcare providers, at (708) 966-5595 for additional information about pain units in your area.

2. *Choose a good program that is convenient for you and your family:*
   - Many pain management programs do not offer outpatient care. Choosing a program close to your home will enable you to commute to the program each day.

3. *Learn something about the people who run the program:*
   - Try to meet several of the staff members to get a sense of the people you will be dealing with while in the unit.

   - The program should have a complete medical staff trained in pain management techniques including:
     - a physician (he or she may be a specialist from a number of different areas but should have expertise in pain management)
     - a registered nurse
     - a psychiatrist or psychologist

---

*The following "Guidelines for Selecting a Pain Management Program" are reproduced by permission of the American Chronic Pain Association, P.O. Box 850, Rocklin, CA 95677.

- a physical therapist
- an occupational therapist
- a biofeedback therapist
- a family counselor
- a vocational counselor
- personnel trained in pain management intervention.

4. *Make sure the program includes most of the following features:*
   - biofeedback training
   - counseling
   - family counseling
   - TENS Units
   - regional anesthesia (nerve blocks)
   - physical therapy (exercise and body mechanics training, hot massage, whirlpool, etc.)
   - relaxation training and stress management
   - educational programs covering medications and other aspects of pain and its management
   - aftercare (follow-up support once you have left the unit)
   - group therapy
   - occupational therapy
   - assertiveness training.

5. *Be sure your family can be involved in your care:*
   - Family members should be required to be involved in your treatment.
   - The program should provide special educational sessions for family members.
   - Joint counseling for you and your family should also be available.

6. *Also consider these additional factors:*
   - What services will your insurance company reimburse, and what will you be expected to cover?
   - What is the unit's physical set-up? (Is it in a patient care area or in an area by itself?)
   - What is the program's length of stay?
   - Is the program inpatient or outpatient (when going through medication detoxification, inpatient care is recommended)
   - If you choose an out-of-town unit, can your family be involved in your care?

- Do you understand what will be required of you during your stay (length of time you will be on unit, responsibility to take care of personal needs, etc.)?
- Does the unit provide any type of job retraining?
- Make sure that, before accepting you, the unit reviews your previous medical records and gives you a complete physical evaluation to be sure you can participate in the program.
- Your personal physician can refer you to the unit, but many programs also accept self-referral.
- Obtain copies of your recent medical records to prevent duplicate testing.
- Try to talk with both present and past program participants to get their feedback about their stay on the unit.

Pain management can make a significant difference in your life; however, you must realize that much of what you gain from your stay will be up to you. Treatment is designed to help you get out of the patient role and back to being a self-sufficient person. The program should help to restore your ability to function and to enjoy life. It will be up to you to become actively involved in the program if you expect to regain control of your life. Pain programs are difficult, but the benefits can improve your lifestyle!

6

Your Weight and Chronic Pain

While few studies confirm that the foods you eat can make a noticeable difference in chronic pain, there are excellent reports showing that weight control and proper nutrition are important for total well-being. It makes sense that if we focus on a diet that is low in fat and high in fiber, vitamins, and nutrients and if we move around more, it will be easier to reap the benefits of achieving optimal weight and feeling energetic.

Statistics show that from 25 to 64 percent of Americans are overweight. For people with chronic pain, staying at a reasonable weight is important for increased energy and flexibility, and for overcoming other problems such as hypertension, diabetes, heart disease, and certain types of cancer—all of which can be influenced by obesity. For people with arthritis or chronic back pain, the more serious the weight problem, the greater is the pressure placed on the back and joints. This can result in more inflammation and increased pain. Just being ten or fifteen pounds overweight can exacerbate a joint or back condition.

What you eat greatly affects the way you feel, and for those who are already suffering with chronic pain, this is an important consideration. Here we will outline the latest dietary recommendations for weight loss and for maintaining a proper weight. If you are not overweight and can stay within a specific weight range, then review this chapter to see if you are doing all you can to help your body stay fit.

EAT FOR GOOD HEALTH

The last thing many people with chronic pain want to be bothered with is another schedule or program. One woman suffering from severe rheumatoid arthritis said, "After I take my medications, do my exercise routine, then do the activities for stress reduction, the last thing I need to worry about is a weight loss program." Another patient told of staying on a very low-calorie diet while trying to lose weight, only to find it didn't work. After going off the diet, she gained back what she had lost plus an additional seven pounds, which is a pattern typical of yo-yo dieting.

This chapter is not about following a weight loss "diet" or a "program." Weight loss diets are not effective for many people, and most programs just don't work. Studies show that approximately 95 percent of people who go on weight loss diets will gain all or some of the weight back within one year. In fact, some studies have found that after a period of five years, not one "advertised" diet program was successful in keeping the weight off.

Instead of a quick fix for weight reduction, why not focus on eating for good health instead of eating to reduce weight? The guidelines we recommend are easy to remember and are consistent with the new Pyramid diet plan advocated by the American Dietetics Association, giving the necessary foods for health in the proper amounts and categories.

HOW'S YOUR COMMITMENT TO A HEALTHY BODY?

Before starting on the road to a healthy body and a healthy outlook, you must first determine if you are ready to make a commitment to permanent change. Changing a lifetime of habits is very difficult to do; there are no shortcuts. It takes commitment, support, motivation, and determination to be successful at weight loss. The following quiz will help determine if you are ready to make lifelong changes.

YES	MAYBE	NO
5 pts.	3 pts.	0 pts.

1. Are you confident that you can make the necessary changes?

2. Do you want control over your health and your chronic pain?

3. Will you be satisfied losing ½ to 1 pound per week?

4. Are you willing to be more physically active?

5. Do you have a social support system of family and friends?

6. Do you have a plan of what you will do instead of overeating?

7. Can you avoid self-blame when you slip up, and can you pick yourself up and continue toward your goals?

YES	NO
0 pts.	5 pts.

8. Have you moved recently?

9. Have you changed jobs recently?

10. Are you recently widowed or divorced?

Add up your score and place the total here _____.

If you scored 35 to 50 points, you are ready to make the changes necessary for permanent weight management. If you scored 20 to 35 points, you are not quite ready to make major, permanent changes at this time. If you continually find excuses for why you can't make the changes, review the questions and see if you can't strengthen your commitment. If you can't, now is not a good time to try.

If you scored 0 to 20 points, there are too many obstacles in your life right now for you to be successful making permanent lifestyle changes. Continue to think of reasons why it would be beneficial to lose weight. When you are ready to make a total commitment, and you have social support and confidence in yourself, then you will be successful. If you try now, you are likely to fail. Remember, yo-yo dieting is worse than being overweight but stable.

NOW LET'S WEIGH IN

Perhaps you have avoided height/weight charts in the past. One fifty-year-old man who has chronic back pain from a football injury said he would never weigh himself again because he didn't weigh the same as he did in college. Remember, charts give only what is "average" for most people. These averages allow women to be "smaller boned" than men. But if you are a small-boned male or a large-boned female, you may be normal at either end of the scale given for your height and age. And it is a waste of energy to try to have the same weight that you did in high school! You cannot change your genetic makeup, but you can change the way you eat.

The height/weight chart (figure 6.1) gives an average weight range for all adults and takes age into consideration. The reason is that the new government guidelines have broader limits than was previously the case: they take into account height, bone structure, and age.

If your weight is a little higher than these figures, then all you might have to do to feel your best is to watch your fat and caloric intake more closely, and move around more. But if your weight is a great deal higher than these figures, then perhaps you should make some careful lifestyle and dietary changes as you seek to lower your weight and lessen your chronic pain. Your physician can recommend a registered dietician to work with you to reduce your weight, and by doing so lessen your chronic pain.

HEIGHT	WEIGHT IN POUNDS	
	19–34 YEARS	**35 YEARS AND OVER**
5'0"	97–128	108–138
5'1"	101–132	111–143
5'2"	104–137	115–148
5'3"	107–141	119–152
5'4"	111–146	122–157
5'5"	114–150	126–162
5'6"	118–155	130–167
5'7"	121–160	134–172
5'8"	125–164	138–178
5'9"	129–169	142–183
5'10"	132–174	146–188
5'11"	136–179	151–194
6'0"	140–184	155–199
6'1"	144–189	159–205
6'2"	148–195	164–210
6'3"	152–200	168–216
6'4"	156–205	173–222
6'5"	160–211	177–228
6'6"	164–216	182–234

NOTE: Height measured without shoes; weight measured without clothes.

Figure 6.1. Suggested weights for adults

HOW MANY CALORIES?

The American Dietetic Association recommends a calorie level of no less than ten times your desired weight, with women getting at least 1200 calories and men getting at least 1400 calories per day. For example, if your goal is to be 140 pounds you should eat around 1400 calories per day. If your goal is 170 pounds, follow a daily diet of 1700 calories. If you follow this recommendation, don't expect to see a quick reduction of weight, but studies show that the chances of gradually losing weight and keeping it off are much greater. And for helping with chronic pain— the kind of pain that is with you day and night—you need long-term assistance with weight management.

Wanda O., a thirty-year-old woman with chronic neck pain, wanted to lose thirty pounds with a weight goal of 140. She told of staying on a low-fat, high complex carbohydrate diet for six weeks, and even began a light walking program. Still, six weeks later, she had gained two pounds instead of losing weight. Finally, her dietician asked Wanda to record her daily food intake for two weeks and come in again.

After two weeks, Wanda brought in a record of what she had been eating every day. Instead of staying at about 1400 calories, Wanda had eaten over 2100 calories. The choices she had made were low-fat and high complex carbohydrates, but she had eaten more calories than her body needed for weight loss. After starting again to record her daily food intake, Wanda could see where she had overindulged and began cutting back while continuing her walking and exercise program. In three months, she had lost fifteen pounds and had changed her eating lifestyle so that the low-fat, high complex carbohydrate dietary changes were natural. The benefits to her of a slimmer waistline and more energy gave her the motivation she needed to continue the new lifestyle of eating and exercise. Without the unnecessary weight bearing on her joints, she felt pain relief.

USE THE NEW FOOD GUIDE PYRAMID

The U.S. Department of Agriculture has designed the new Food Guide Pyramid as an excellent guideline for calculating a healthy diet (see figure 6.2). As you follow the Pyramid plan shown, make most of your food choices from the widest part, or the pyramid bottom, and use the top part of the Pyramid sparingly.

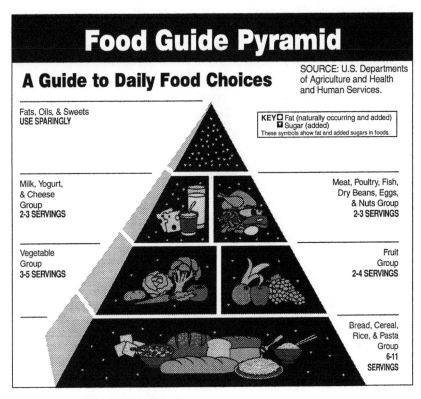

Food Guide Pyramid

A Guide to Daily Food Choices

SOURCE: U.S. Departments of Agriculture and Health and Human Services.

Fats, Oils, & Sweets
USE SPARINGLY

KEY☐ Fat (naturally occurring and added)
▼ Sugar (added)
These symbols show fat and added sugars in foods.

Milk, Yogurt,
& Cheese
Group
2-3 SERVINGS

Meat, Poultry, Fish,
Dry Beans, Eggs,
& Nuts Group
2-3 SERVINGS

Vegetable
Group
3-5 SERVINGS

Fruit
Group
2-4 SERVINGS

Bread, Cereal,
Rice, & Pasta
Group
6-11
SERVINGS

Figure 6.2. The Food Guide Pyramid: A guide to daily food choices

WEIGHT REDUCTION AND MAINTENANCE

1. Reduce Fat

Reducing fat may be the easiest and most healthful way to reduce your weight and control your chronic pain. Instead of eating like a bird, eating low-fat foods including vegetables, fruits, breads, whole grain cereals, legumes, fish, and skinless chicken will allow you to feel full and still lose weight.

High-fat diets should be a great concern for most people, accounting for 40 to 50 percent of the total calories in a "typical" American diet, at a time when government guidelines recommend no more than 30 percent of calories from fat for good health. A diet high in fat has been attributed to certain types of diseases, including heart disease and certain types of cancers.

Fat can be easily recognizable in your diet in foods such as potato chips, hamburgers and fries, and a bacon and egg breakfast. But some fats are dangerously hidden in such seemingly healthy foods as oatmeal and raisin bars, peanut butter, some yogurt, popcorn cooked in oil, granola, and more.

The recommendation for everyone is to limit fat to less than 30 percent of the total intake of calories each day. Some healthcare professionals ask patients to lower their fat intake to 20 percent of the total intake of calories each day, or even lower. While this low amount of fat in the daily diet seems out of reach, it can be done easily by making some substitutions in your daily diet: replacing whole milk with skim milk, butter with reduced-fat margarine, regular yogurt with no-fat yogurt, fried chicken with baked skinless chicken, and fried chips with baked low-salt crackers (see table 6.1 for more ways to reduce fat).

Table 6.1. Ways to reduce fat in your diet

Change This	To This
ice cream	ice milk, sherbet, frozen yogurt
butter	no-fat or reduced-fat margarine
whole milk	low-fat or skimmed milk
creamed soups	low-fat variety and skimmed milk
french fries	baked oven fries
potato chips	baked crackers or pretzels
cream	evaporated skim milk
fried chicken	baked chicken without skin
spaghetti sauce with meat	spaghetti with tomato sauce
hamburger	chicken sandwich
candy bar	fudgsicle
grilled cheese sandwich	grilled cheese sandwich with no-fat cheese
chocolate candy	no-fat jelly beans or candy corn
omelet	egg substitutes or egg whites
pancakes, biscuits, muffins	bagels, English muffins, rice cakes
chocolate chip cookies	fig bars, gingersnaps
pound cake	angel food cake
regular mayonnaise	low-fat or no-fat mayonnaise

Table 6.1 (cont.)

Change This	**To This**
tartar sauce	cocktail sauce or salsa
cream cheese on bagel	no-fat cream cheese on bagel

How do you know if a product is high or low in fat? *Read the label!* Package labels include the ingredients, the calories, the nutrients, the sodium, and much more for the consumer's information (see table 6.2 for a sample label).

Table 6.2. Sample Label

Clam Chowder

Ingredients: clam broth, potatoes, tomato paste, carrots, clams, celery, sweet peppers, modified food starch, salt, vegetable oil (corn, cottonseed, or partially hydrogenated soybean oil), water, wheat flour, monosodium glutamate, dehydrated parsley, natural flavoring, yeast extract, and spice.

Nutritional Information Per Serving

Serving size:	4 oz.
Servings per container:	2¾
Calories:	70
Protein (grams):	2
Carbohydrate (grams):	10
Fat (grams):	2
Cholesterol:	less than 5 mg/serving
Sodium:	820 mg/serving

After reading the label, you can figure out if this is a high, moderate, or low-fat food by using the following formula:

1 gram fat = 9 calories
If the serving has 2 grams of fat, then
$2 \times 9 = 18$ calories from fat.
If the total calories of the serving are 100, then:
$18/100 = 18\%$ of calories from fat.

This food would be considered a low-fat food with under 20 percent of fat calories.

Table 6.3. Know your fats

Saturated fat: fat that comes from animal and whole milk dairy products; also from some oils (examples: red meat, butter, cheeses, luncheon meats, coconut oil, palm oil, cream).

Unsaturated fat: fat that is usually a liquid. It is not as bad for you as saturated fats.

Monounsaturated fat: fat that comes from plant foods, including canola and olive oils.

Polyunsaturated fat: fat that is found in plants, including sunflower, corn, soybean, and safflower oils.

Table 6.4. Guidelines to reduce fat

- Keep your fat intake to 30 percent or less of your daily caloric intake

- Choose no-fat or low-fat food items

- Stay away from foods high in saturated fats (no more than 10 percent per day)

- No more than 10 percent of your calories should come from *polyunsaturated* fat

- Ten to fifteen percent of your calories should come from *mono-unsaturated* fat

- Fill up on complex carbohydrates (starch and fiber)

- Eat five servings of vegetables per day instead of high-fat choices.

Calculating Fat Calories

Trying to stay below 30 percent fat calories each day means that you must carefully calculate this amount. After several weeks of doing this, it will become a "low-fat habit," and you will naturally turn to the healthier foods instead of unhealthy fat choices.

If you eat 1500 calories each day, you can calculate your fat calories by using the following formula:

1500 calories × 30 percent fat calories = 450 calories from fat.

You can now determine how many grams of fat are allowed per day:

450 calories from fat / 9 calories per gram of fat = 50 grams of fat per day.

2. Increase Fiber and Complex Carbohydrates

Fiber and complex carbohydrates are said to be nature's "miracle" foods. Not only do complex carbohydrates fill us up so we don't indulge on high-fat snacks, the fiber keeps our system running and regular. Research has shown that people who eat a diet high in fiber have a lower incidence of colon cancer, the second most common cancer in America. While the National Cancer Institute recommends eating 20 to 35 grams of fiber each day, the average person eats less than 15 grams.

There are different types of fiber. *Soluble fiber* is found in oats, fruits, vegetables, and legumes. This type of fiber helps to lower blood cholesterol and maintain blood sugar. *Insoluble fiber* is found in wheats, bran, and whole grains. Insoluble fiber is good for the digestive system and may offer protection against certain cancers.

You can increase your dietary fiber and lower your risk of some cancers by adding at least six servings of breads, cereals, pasta, rice, dried peas, and beans and two to four servings of fresh, frozen, canned or dried fruits and three to five servings of vegetables. As you begin to choose low-fat, high complex carbohydrate foods in your diet, you can gradually notice a reduction in your weight. For most people with chronic pain, this is an appreciated added benefit as it means less weight to cause increased stress on the painful back or joints (see table 6.5 for the fiber content of common foods).

Table 6.5. Fiber content of common foods

	Amount	*Grams*
Breads		
bagel	1 bagel	1
bran	1 slice	3
cornbread	1 piece	1.3
English muffin (wheat)	1	2
white	1 slice	1
wheat	1 slice	2
Cereals		
Fiber One	1 ounce	12
All Bran	1 ounce	9
grits, uncooked	¼ cup	4.9
Life	1 ounce	2
Corn flakes	1 ounce	1
Cocoa Krispies	1 ounce	0
waffle	1	0.5
Fruits		
apple with skin	1 medium	3
banana	1 medium	1.5
grapes	½ cup	.7
orange	1 medium	3.8
pear	1 medium	4.5
raspberries	1 cup	6.0
strawberries	1¼ cup	6.5
watermelon	1¼ cup	1.75
Fruits (Dried)		
apricots	5 halves	6.0
figs	1½	4.5
prunes, medium	3	4
raisins	2 tbsp.	1.2
Vegetables		
beans, green	½ cup	1.5
broccoli, cooked	½ cup	1.1
cabbage, cooked	½ cup	1.5

Table 6.5 (cont.)

	Amount	*Grams*
carrots, raw	1 medium	3.7
corn	½ cup	3.2
cauliflower	1 cup raw	3.6
kidney beans (red)	1 cup	15
lettuce	1 cup	1
lima beans	½ cup	4.8
potato, baked with skin	1 medium	3.5
potato, sweet	1 medium	7.3

Table 6.6. Guidelines to increase fiber

- Eat more legumes that are very high in fiber: red beans, black beans, great northern beans and other legumes are high in fiber and have no fat. (Be careful, though: don't cook them with animal fat!)

- Eat raw vegetables for snacks. Two carrots will give you a day's supply of vitamin A and provide over seven grams of fiber.

- Read your cereal box at the grocery. If the cereal has no fiber or less than three grams, it probably has little nutrient value.

- Add dried fruits to your cereal. Three prunes can give you four grams of fiber.

- Keep your vegetables crisp when you cook them instead of soft. Eat these with skins on to add to the fiber content.

3. Move Around More

While moving around more is not a dietary change, it is a necessary lifestyle change if you expect to notice any difference in your weight and your energy level. Moving around does not mean that you have to go out and run for miles; for many people with chronic pain, this is out of the question anyway. But moving around does mean that you make an effort throughout the day to get up and walk around, bend down and touch your toes, wave your arms, walk, twist, skip, or make your body move in some way—without adding to your pain.

Exercise is important in the prevention of some types of chronic pain: not only is the body strengthened but you add flexibility and increased circulation. Researchers now recommend at least thirty minutes a day of movement exercise for good health. Those with chronic pain might have to do this five or ten minutes at a time until they become accustomed to increased activity, but make it a goal to be active for at least thirty minutes every day.

In chapter 4, exercises are offered to increase the strength and mobility of persons with chronic pain. Perform these exercises daily along with maintaining the low-fat, high complex carbohydrate eating plan for good health. You will notice a difference in the way you look and, more importantly, in the way you feel.

Table 6.7. Ways to burn calories with activity

Activity	Minutes to burn 100 calories
bicycling	26 (6 mph.)
cleaning house	27
cooking meals	37
dancing	34 (slow)
dancing	12 (fast)
dusting	41
ironing	53
jogging	13 (5 mph.)
mowing lawn (power)	29
stationary cycling	16 (10 mph.)
swimming	30
typing	59
vacuuming	19
walking	27 (3 mph.)
walking	18 (4 mph.)
washing windows	29
watching television	79

4. Keep a Food Diary

As you start your lifestyle plan of diet and exercise to help end chronic pain, keep a food diary. Studies have shown that when obese people are asked to record their daily food intake in order to maintain a low-fat, low-calorie diet, the results are surprising. The same people who said they ate no more than 1100 calories and 20 percent fat calories per day, topped off at an average of over 2000 calories and with 60 percent fat calories per day. *This made a tremendous difference that resulted in weight gain instead of loss!*

Keeping a food diary helps you know exactly where you stand nutritionally. You may think you are eating a low-fat diet, but after calculating your fats at the end of the day, you find that you have eaten over 40 percent in fat calories. Or you may think you are getting between 20 and 35 grams of fiber each day, when, in fact, you are getting only 9 grams.

Until you get in the "good health habit," keeping a food diary will help keep you organized and honest! Use it as you would a check book, putting your daily calories, fat, and fiber grams in the spaces indicated. As you go through the day, calculate the amount of nutrients and calories in your diet. If you are over the amount in calories and fats, make adjustments the next day. The diary is a good indicator of what you really eat.

Copy the sample food diaries on pp. 170–171 in a notebook, and use these to stick with your eating plan for good health. Don't be hard on yourself, but use this as a learning and awareness tool. We have filled in one meal for you to use as a sample.

Once you have a record of your current eating habits, you can begin to change those things you need to. Using the following questionnaire you will be able to determine specific changes you need to make.

Eating Style Profile

Questions   (Answer with: YES   NO   SOMETIMES)

1. Do you overeat when you are angry?
2. Do you try every new diet that comes out?
3. Do you rush through your meals without tasting each bite?
4. Do you find it unbearable if you run out of your favorite foods or snacks?
5. Could you always eat dessert even after a four-course meal?
6. Do you continue eating even when you are full?
7. Do you like to eat no matter what food tastes like?
8. Do you eat when you are sad or depressed?
9. Do you make a shopping list for the supermarket and ignore it if something looks appealing?
10. Do you think of food even when you are not eating?
11. Do you use added fats and oils to your foods?

12. Do you engage in unrelated activities, such as reading, paperwork, watching TV, etc., while you are eating?
13. Do you keep tempting foods around your kitchen or in the refrigerator?
14. Do you overeat when you are comfortable and relaxed?
15. Do you eat to take your mind off your worries?
16. Do you enjoy sweets and alcohol each day?
17. Have you ever eaten food and not remembered eating it?
18. Do you go off your diet completely during holidays and vacations?
19. Do you overeat when you are happy?
20. Do you lack the support of family and friends?
21. When you slip from your diet, do you give up?
22. Do you binge?
23. Do you starve yourself to lose weight?
24. Do you get anxious or angry if someone else gets more food?
25. Do you hide food or snacks in your home or at work?
26. Do you eat even when you are not hungry?
27. Are your food portions too large?
28. Do you eat constantly all day long?
29. Do you skip meals?
30. Am you a member of the clean plate club?
31. Do you eat a lot of high-fat, high-calorie foods?
32. Are there certain foods you cannot stop eating once you have begun?
33. Do you reward yourself with food?
34. Does the sight or smell of certain foods trigger the desire to eat?
35. Do certain places trigger the desire to eat?
36. Do you go grocery shopping when you are hungry?
37. Do you overeat when you am bored?
38. Do you make yourself vomit if you feel full?

After completion, look over the questionnaire. If you checked "No" on most questions, then your eating habits are probably in control. But if your answers were "Sometimes" or "Yes," you have some work to do.

As you check your questionnaire, do you see a pattern with your eating habits? Are you a binger or do you sneak food late at night? Do you eat high-fat foods or do you nibble on sweets all day? From your answers, you can begin to set specific goals for change. Start with those questions you marked "Sometimes," since those goals will be more easily attainable. Make your goals realistic and be flexible. Do not attempt immediately to change something you know will be very difficult for you to alter. By starting with easier changes, you will be able to feel successful. If you attempt a change you are not ready for, you may set yourself up for failure.

IT'S UP TO YOU!

Starting and maintaining a low-fat, high complex carbohydrate weight control program may not be easy at first. Making plans to become more active, including starting the daily exercise program outlined in chapter 4, may well be a difficult lifestyle change. But studies show that people who stay on low-fat diets over six months or more find that their tastes gravitate toward foods that are naturally low in fat. And people who begin exercising start to look forward to it after a few weeks.

This chapter offers you some basic suggestions on how to begin eating and moving for good health. Take these ideas and implement them in your diet today. As you plan your weekly menu, make low-fat, high complex carbohydrate choices. And, most important, don't keep foods around your kitchen that invite you to fail.

It's up to you! Winning with chronic pain will involve some drastic lifestyle changes that only you can make. But the rewards of being able to lead an active, normal life are well worth the sacrifice.

Food Diary (sample)				
Day/Food	Amount	Fats	Fiber	Calories
Monday				
Breakfast				
egg	1 medium	5.1	0	75
wheat bread	2 slices	2	4	150
strawberry jelly	1 tbsp.	0	0	30
skim milk	8 ounces	0	0	80
prunes	3	1	4	75

Food Diary (sample)

Day   *Calories and/or Fat Grams*

Breakfast Time:

Lunch Time:

Dinner Time:

Snacks Times:

Feelings/comments/exercise:

At the end of each week, make an assessment of what you have accomplished. You can copy and use the form on the following page.

Weekly Weight Control Assessment

Date: Weight:

Average Caloric Intake:

Average Fat Gram Intake:

Measurements: Chest/Bust: Waist:

                  Hips: Thighs:

Exercise   *Activity*

Monday—

Tuesday—

Wednesday—

Thursday—

Friday—

Saturday—

Sunday—

Goals Worked on This Week:

Helpful Strategies Used:

Goals for Next Week:

7

Coping with Chronic Pain

If your chronic pain has lasted for months, it could feel like an eternity. In fact, the pain may have been with you for so long and have been so debilitating that you have difficulty remembering what it was like to live without pain. When, for example, the chronic back pain, headache, or nerve pain started, you thought there would be an end to the suffering, and you may have tried every medical solution that any doctor or friend recommended. You may also have sought psychological help, not because you thought the pain was "all in your head," but because you were experiencing anxiety, fearfulness, depression, exhaustion, insomnia, irritability, or other problems.

COPING WITH STAYING WELL

When staying well is mentioned to people with chronic pain, they may have thoughts of the physical determinants of health: exercise, diet, heredity, relaxation, and avoidance of unhealthy habits, such as smoking. Recently, however, the psychological and social makeup of people has been recognized as highly influential in determining the condition of their health. The area of study showing the most promise is a personality trait researchers call *hardiness*. Hardy people have fewer and less severe illnesses. Hardy people are able to deal with chronic pain and move on to an active and productive life.

WHO IS A HARDY INDIVIDUAL?

Hardy people are those who anticipate change with excitement. They view change as a challenge rather than as a threat. They are open and

173

flexible, exhibit optimism, reappraise their assumptions when events seem inconsistent with their beliefs, and are more successful in obtaining help.

How Does a Person with Chronic Pain Become Hardy?

Control, commitment, and *challenge* are necessary for developing hardiness. *Control* refers to feeling "in control" of the major areas of life even when you are in chronic pain. Hardy people *know* that if they lose their job or their marriage ends or if they lose control of certain areas of their life, they will survive the trauma. When a problem occurs, hardy people initially blame themselves for situations that have gone sour in their lives but will then find ways to change their behavior and take action. They *maintain* their sense of control and face future stressful situations with determination rather than helplessness.

Commitment means being involved rather than alienated. Hardy people approach life with a sense of purpose and take the action necessary to remedy difficult situations. When it comes to health, hardy people who experience chronic pain make a commitment to themselves and set their own limits. They make healthy habits a priority and consider change when an environment becomes destructive to their resolve.

Challenge refers to facing change with an attitude of determination. It involves taking action to change either oneself or one's situation in an effort to become healthy. Some people with chronic pain allow fear to halt their efforts, but hardy people press on despite the fear.

Why aren't we all hardy individuals? Is it possible for someone with constant, unending pain to consider being well and hardy? The primary obstacle is centered on how we *interpret* problems in our lives. One research study* set out to demonstrate how powerful an influence interpretation can be: seventy-five-year-olds were placed in a retreat center for one week and were told to "be fifty-five again." The center was retrofitted with surroundings (even telephones and magazines) from twenty years earlier. After one week, their hearing, eyesight, dexterity, and appetites improved. Their mental ability also improved, and they stood physically taller!

What people believe actually influences whether action or inaction takes place in their lives. To take positive action in the face of difficulty (e.g., divorce, job loss, or death), it is essential to reexamine what you believe and why. This reappraisal of one's belief system is done naturally by hardy individuals, even those in chronic pain. The rest of us need

---

*Ellen J. Langer, *Mindfulness* (Reading, Mass.: Addison-Wesley, 1990).

assistance and usually get it by seeking counsel. With sufficient counseling, people do reassess their thinking and take the necessary action to promote a healthy life.

SURVIVAL SKILLS FOR HARDY LIVING

Control

- Reevaluate your beliefs about a difficult situation.

- Reassess the situation.

- Make decisions (do not just "ride the tide").

- Take responsibility for your decisions.

- Understand how much you control your life, including your health and the pain.

- Determine and set your own limits.

Commitment

- Get involved in something you believe in.

- Combat guilt.

- Surround yourself with positive people.

- Make a commitment to yourself. ("I *will* take care of me!" "I *will* never allow that to devastate me again!")

- Maintain healthy habits.

- Consider change when the environment is destructive to your commitment.

Challenge

- Look for growth and opportunity in change.

- Consult with others and draw on their experience.

- Take one step at a time.

- Make a plan.

- Use your reason to moderate and channel self-destructive and negative feelings.

- Use humor to help you through.

- Make a conscious effort to see the good in the world.

CHRONIC PAIN INVOLVES THE WHOLE PERSON

As you work toward becoming a "hardy" individual in the midst of unending pain, you must confront a variety of emotions and behaviors experienced by people with chronic pain, including back pain, osteoporosis, arthritis, headache, neck pain, nerve pain, the pain of cancer, and the like. You may recognize yourself in all these discussions, or you may think that only a few apply to you. In any event, it would be good to read about all the areas, just in case you experience a problem later and can then recall some suggestions put forth. Each emotion or behavior experience by persons with chronic pain is addressed in two ways:

(1) a brief description of the feeling or behavior, and

(2) personal strategies or suggestions for helping you cope with each situation.

If you have accepted the fact that you may have to live with some degree of pain for a long period, maybe even a lifetime, you will be better able to benefit from the suggested techniques. It is no fun to be in pain, and at times you may have expressed the sentiment that "A life with pain is no life at all." Your problems are very real, and they often have a devastating affect on your outlook on life and on your daily activities. By going through each of the negative areas, you can develop very effective strategies for coping with them for better enjoyment of life.

Read each of the following coping and survival strategies with an open mind: you *can* have an impact on your own life. There are areas you can change, and there are definite alternatives to relying on medical intervention.

Acceptance

As a chronic pain patient, your ultimate goal is to get to the point where you can accept the pain, then be ready to make modifications to handle it in your life. The opposite of acceptance is denial. Denial is the behavior that works against pain rehabilitation efforts. It is vital to accept the fact that nonmedical issues such as suspiciousness, anxiety, anger, or loss of self-esteem can and do affect your pain. If you are not willing to admit this, you will have no reason to engage in any type of rehabilitation therapy.

Denial or nonacceptance is often the way you preserve your self-esteem. You may think that if you admit that anything other than a physical problem is increasing your pain, your friends and family will think that the pain is not physical but psychological or the product of your imagination. This is certainly not the case. Stress factors in the family or even at work can affect all areas of your life: your thoughts, your outlook on life, and, yes, even your pain. Acceptance is the first step in successful rehabilitation.

Survival Strategies for Reaching Acceptance

1. *Keep your mind open to nonmedical treatment.* A variety of treatments, such as relaxation and biofeedback, are available and can easily be learned. These stress managers really do work! See the relaxation response in chapter 5 for an example and practice it daily until you are able to use this tool when you feel anxious.

2. *Do not feel that because you are seeing a counselor your friends or family members will think the pain is something you imagined.* Psychological intervention can often bring relief of chronic pain when medical treatment has failed. How you react to stressors in your life can be helped with a qualified therapist as you learn positive coping skills.

3. *Keep a daily record of your feelings and the intensity of your pain.* Ask a counselor or your doctor to look at this diary and help you work through the painful moments by changing negative behaviors or actions.

4. *Accept your chronic pain.* This does not mean that you have to "like" the pain, but acceptance will allow you to redirect your life as you begin to manage the pain. As you begin coping techniques and the medical treatment plan, you will experience lessened pain, which will be an unanticipated benefit.

Coping with Constant Anxiety and Fears

Every chronic pain patient experiences feelings of anxiety and fear, which can be very real, and usually involve questions about the future:

- Will my pain become unbearable?

- Can I handle it if the pain increases?

- Will I become homebound?

- Will my friends leave me alone with my pain?

- Will I be able to keep my job?

- How can I wake up each day if it worsens?

- Will I be able to care for my family?

Becoming obsessive about your fears—dwelling on what may happen—will make it difficult to move in a positive direction. It is far better to recognize your fears and redirect your energy toward optimistic behaviors in order to stop or change negative thoughts and actions. Worrying about what cannot be changed will only make you more anxious and fearful.

Survival Strategies for Ending Anxiety and Fears

1. *Write down on paper the very situations that make you anxious and fearful.* These may include a certain program or newscast on television, the negative response of a friend, conflict with a family member who does not accept your chronic pain, or even reading the morning paper. Try to avoid these situations when possible so you are not confronted with fearful areas.

2. *Do not expect your family or friends to be your therapists.* Find a licensed mental health counselor and make an appointment to "talk it out" with an impartial trained professional who understands the problems of those who suffer with pain.

3. *Broaden your views on nontraditional therapies.* Keep an open mind about nonmedical interventions that can help you relax, such as biofeedback, relaxation response, music therapy, and the like.

4. *Join a support group of chronic pain patients.* See chapter 5 for groups across the United States that are open to people with chronic

pain. If there is no support group in your area, ask for instructions on how to start one. Take the initiative and help yourself.

5. *Ask your doctor to explain the nature of chronic pain to your family.* Most particularly, have him explain why there are some days when you do better than other days. This will help your family to become more understanding and empathic when your pain is severe.

Coping with Suspicion

Living with chronic pain can make you more sensitive to the thoughts and actions of others. Constant, unrelenting pain day after day can result in distorted thoughts and behavior. This does not mean that you are crazy. Instead, it means that the stress has affected the way you interpret what people do and say.

If you find yourself being overly suspicious, sit back and consider the possibility that you might be overreacting. Ask a trusted friend or counselor about your accusations, but be sure you are going to listen to the response and not berate the person for having a different opinion.

No one is asking you to be naive about people and their motives. Instead, you should realize that living in pain is stressful enough to distort your thinking.

Survival Strategies for Suspiciousness

1. Relearn to trust others.

2. Even if people are doing and saying things you don't like, try not let it bother you to the point of not accepting their word.

3. Confront those involved with your suspicions. If they have a reasonable response, believe them.

4. Remember that harboring negative thoughts about others (even if such thoughts are true) is detrimental to your health and general outlook on life.

5. Look carefully at the people who arouse your suspicion, and see if there is an alternative explanation for their actions.

Coping with Anger and Irritability

Anger is a natural reaction to chronic pain, but how one responds to the anger can vary. Some use the anger in a positive manner, others ignore it, and still others let angry feelings consume their whole being. In order to cope with the anger and irritability that often accompanies chronic pain, it will help to try and understand these feelings better. Once you do this, you can replace the energy you spend being angry with positive actions to make your life enjoyable for you and those around you.

If you have lived with unending chronic pain for months or years, you definitely have a right to be angry, but you do not have a right to hurt yourself and others while expressing this anger.

Survival Strategies for Anger and Irritability

1. Anger is an emotion that can destroy your health if not expressed in a positive manner. It is important to realize that anger can contribute to the pain you're experiencing.

2. Anger is an emotion that everyone is entitled to feel at times; but again, it is important to express this in a way that will not be detrimental to your overall health and well-being, nor to those around you.

3. If anger is consuming your entire day, realize that you need to find some avenues for changing this.

4. If your anger gets out of control on a "bad" day, stop immediately and apologize to those around you.

5. Write down on paper the very situations or persons who create angry feelings in you. Try to avoid getting into these situations if you feel you might explode.

6. Ask your doctor to recommend a professional who can give you some tools for coping with angry feelings.

Coping with Loss of Control

In addition to feelings of anger and irritability, chronic pain can cause loss of control over other aspects of your life. You may have noticed that those facets of life that once depended on your abilities, ideas, or strength no longer do. Instead of being in control of your destiny, you may feel that the pain controls every aspect of your life; you are simply a puppet on a string.

There is a fine line between what you *think* you cannot control and what you *absolutely* cannot control. The key to dealing effectively with pain is to make sure you understand this distinction.

Survival Strategies for Loss of Control

1. *Make a list of the things you want to change in your life.* With the help of your doctor, mental health counselor, family, and friends, start applying yourself to the areas in your life that you still have control over.

2. *Learn to adjust.* If you are no longer able to work and must give it up, do not get stressed over the situation. Talk to someone about your feelings and fears, and learn to channel these feelings in another direction that you *do* have some control over.

3. *Ask for help.* If you need help with an area that you have lost control over, such as cleaning your home or driving to the doctor, ask for assistance. It is not a sign of personal failure to get help from anyone; we all need help at some time in our lives.

4. *Set goals each day to tackle a new area that you have lost control over.* Perhaps you have been unable to clean the house due to chronic pain. Start with one room and try to tackle one project; for example, washing the dishes instead of trying to clean the entire kitchen. As you accomplish one project, weigh the amount of pain you are experiencing. If you can continue, try another small task. Soon you may be able to regain control over some areas that were isolated by the pain.

5. *Take baby steps in achieving control again.* Remember, taking one small step at a time, then another and another, will let you regain control and confidence over the areas in your life that have been out of reach for some time.

Coping with Avoidance Behaviors

From the time we are infants, we learn to avoid painful actions. If we touched a hot grill and were burned, we learned to stay clear of hot grills. It is natural to want to avoid pain. Until recently, it was considered the right thing to do.

Now that you are experiencing chronic pain, the whole scenario changes. If you constantly avoid the pain, you will become inactive, which increases your chances of keeping and increasing the chronic pain. Does this sound like a vicious circle? It is! You *must* permit yourself to experience the pain in order to get better. All these avoidance behaviors are not helping, at least not in the long run. In behaving this way, you only get short-term relief for long-term pain.

Survival Strategies for Reducing Avoidance Behaviors

1. Make yourself perform at least one activity a day that you would have avoided in the past.

2. Force yourself to participate in one leisure activity a week with family or friends.

3. Never ask anyone else to do something for you what you are capable of doing for yourself.

Coping with Social Isolation

Social isolation may be a three-faceted problem for those in pain. On the one hand, you are purposefully avoiding some people due to fatigue, irritability, pain, or the many other problems you have to face each day. You find your home a secure haven where you are not on display and where there are loved ones around to meet your needs. On the other hand, there may be friends who are purposefully avoiding you. It is possible that you have driven them away by continually focusing on your physical problems. They may be kind and ask about your health, but long lectures on your latest surgery or current pain are not what friends willingly want to hear over and over again.

Moreover, for some people, leaving the bed or house can be associated with wellness. As we explained earlier, you may be fearful that some people who see you "out and about" may assume you are back to "normal." Once you are considered better, family and friends may be quick to expect you to do things that you are actually not capable of doing.

Survival Strategies for Social Isolation

1. Look for nonverbal cues that suggest people are tuning you out as you talk about your pain.

2. Limit pain-related conversations to five minutes.

3. Never turn your back on true friends. They constitute an important support system.

4. When people ask "How are you feeling today?" do not mistake this for an interest in hearing details about how bad you feel.

5. Make yourself go on at least one outing each weekend and one during the week—more if possible, but no less than one each week. This outing may be a trip to the mall, a visit to a friend, or even a walk at a local park.

Coping with Self-Centeredness

When someone goes into the hospital for surgery, family members focus on helping until the patient is up and about again. The same thing happens with a person in pain. However, if the pain goes on for months or years, some patients continue to expect everyone's life to revolve around theirs, and some families continue to provide this attention. It is difficult to change this pattern once it becomes routine. Very few persons approached pain with the idea that they would become self-centered. Nevertheless, you may have fallen into a pattern of focusing solely on yourself. It is easy to do when all thoughts and actions revolve around you.

If this routine has occurred in your home, do not place blame on either side. Instead, talk with your family and begin to initiate changes that are more family-oriented.

Coping Strategies for Changing a Self-Centered Orientation

1. Eliminate certain statements from your interactions with others:
   (a) "My problems are the worst."
   (b) "No one knows the pain I feel."
   (c) "If this ever happens to you, you'll be sorry for how you've treated me."

2. Take time each day to focus on the problem of someone else in your family.

3. Do not let your family focus entirely on your problem.

4. In social situations, try to eliminate all reference to your pain.

5. If there is a difference of opinion as to whether or not you have become self-centered, consider family therapy to iron out the variance in viewpoints.

Coping with Communication Problems

How is it that your family says you never hear what they say, or hear it incorrectly? The most common reasons for misunderstandings in communication are due to other issues, some of which are:

> (1) not listening well because your mind is overrun with worries and fears;
> (2) not focusing on what a person is saying, because of your physical condition (such as being in a lot of pain);
> (3) misinterpreting what is said because your concentration is affected by the pain and related factors (e.g., lack of sleep).

Being in constant pain can easily take your mind off the subject of any conversation. You may actually have gotten into the habit of not listening, thinking that whatever is said will come up again later.

Moreover, you may be experiencing memory problems due to lack of attention and reduced levels of concentration. Though you may be experiencing some or all of these problems, it is very important that you work to keep open and clear lines of communication with your family and loved ones. If they feel that you are not listening to them (for whatever reason), they will be less inclined to listen to you.

Survival Strategies for Communication Problems

1. *Listen* to others when they speak.

2. Ask questions if you are not clear about the details of what is being said.

3. Be direct. Do not just assume, for example, that others will automatically know that you do not want company on the weekend.

4. Avoid indirect communication or body language such as grimaces, slamming doors, sarcasm, or pouting.

5. Consider a community education course on "Enhancing Communication Skills." Check with your local community health center for dates and times.

6. Consider family and/or marital counseling to help improve your communication system in the home.

Coping with Abuse to the Family

You know that your family is most important to you, but it seems that you treat them worse than outsiders. Why is that? Through the years you have always been able to "let down your hair" at home. When you felt bad, it was acceptable to let your family members know. Your family would understand and make allowances for you. However, now that you feel bad almost every day, it is not appropriate to continue to take things out on your loved ones day after day.

Survival Strategies for Abuse to Family

1. Try putting your family above outsiders and yourself.

2. On one day, try pretending your family members are guests and treat them as such.

3. Monitor your angry responses and try to redirect your anger.

4. Apologies are greatly appreciated. Do not assume that your family will know you are feeling remorseful.

5. Remember, when the chips are down, your family members are the ones who will be there. Do not drive them away.

Coping with Stress

Stress can affect most of us, but people with chronic pain are particularly vulnerable to this problem. "Stressed out" is a term used to describe the impact that life stressors have on you. These include anxiety, tension, high blood pressure, depression, anger, distractibility, disorientation, and an entire host of physical problems, but particularly an increase in pain. As a pain sufferer, you experience stressors across all aspects of your life. There are physical stressors (the pain itself), social stressors (loss of friends and activities), work stressors (loss of a job or difficulty working), and family stressors (feelings of dependency on others).

You have every right to be stressed, but this doesn't mean you can do nothing about it.

Survival Strategies for Decreasing Stress

1. Write down the very things that make you "stressed," including situations, people, and the like. Make a conscious effort to avoid the things that you have no control over. For example, an aggressive neighbor who does not believe you have chronic pain should be avoided if this person causes added anxiety.

2. If you are experiencing any physical symptoms of stress, such as high blood pressure, headaches, or anxiety attacks, be sure to consult your physician.

3. Take a class on stress management offered through your community schools or local wellness programs.

4. A therapist who specializes in stress management can help you learn ways of dealing with overwhelming problems, people, and situations.

5. Relaxation tapes are available at local bookstores or learn how to do the relaxation response outlined in chapter 5. Use this type of therapy when you feel your body becoming tense.

Coping with Drug and Alcohol Abuse

Drugs and alcohol are known to decrease pain to some degree; however, their effects are often short-lived and, in addition, you can be left with the pain and the complicated side affects of addiction, depression, and possibly confusion.

When pain first develops, a physician probably will prescribe a narcotic of some type to relieve the acute pain. This is a good way of giving the body some short-term relief in order to heal. However, if the pain lingers and develops into a chronic or long-standing condition, these same drugs are not appropriate or effective. The reason is that the body builds up a tolerance for the drug and it loses its effect— more and more is needed to obtain the same degree of relief received with a lesser dosage.

Alcohol, too, is a substance that requires more and more to dull the discomfort of chronic pain. In addition, it is a depressant that leaves the drinker in a "down" mood once the effects wear off. Long-term use of alcohol also carries with it the danger of cognitive deficits such as memory difficulties, visual and spatial problems, and decreased motor function. It is not a smart trade-off.

In essence, drugs and alcohol are dangerous methods of pain control.

Some drugs may be of value, but you should make sure they are ones that are effective for chronic pain, not acute short-term pain.

Survival Strategies for Drug and Alcohol Abuse

1. If you think that you might be abusing drugs or alcohol, shed your pride and seek professional help.

2. If your family has been asking you to see somebody for the problem, do them and yourself a favor—accept the help.

3. Consult a physician about locating a chronic pain management program in your community.

4. If you believe that you are addicted, consider admitting yourself to the detox section of a pain management inpatient unit in your area.

Coping with Depression

The debilitating effects of depression are ruining the lives of thousands of people with chronic pain. Perhaps you don't feel depressed, but this does not mean you're not experiencing depression. Depressive symptoms can include:

- disturbances in sleep patterns
- loss of interest in daily activities
- weight loss or gain (more than 5 percent of body weight)
- fatigue
- impaired thinking processes
- thoughts of dying or suicide
- mood swings and motivation
- loss of interest in special activities such as hobbies
- staying at home all the time
- avoidance of special friends
- excessive sleep or insomnia
- reduced or increased appetite
- difficulty concentrating.

Some people with chronic pain, however, may be well aware that they are depressed. The signs are obvious: uncontrollable tearfulness, feelings of helplessness and/or hopelessness, loss of self-worth, and suicidal thoughts or plans. If you have these feelings, please contact a professional to get help.

Survival Strategies for Combating Depression

1. See a qualified mental health specialist if depression is immobilizing you.

2. If you have suicidal thoughts, let someone help you. Never keep these thoughts to yourself.

3. Alcohol and drugs cannot combat depression. Use medication only if it is prescribed by your physician.

4. Exercise is a great cure for easing depression. Determine what you can do physically and start getting active.

5. Stick to a routine each day—even when you are in pain. Staying in bed all day, unless advised by your doctor, will not help you alleviate your depressive feelings.

Coping with Loss of Self-Esteem

Chronic pain can affect the pride you have in yourself. It often leads to job loss, decreased contact with friends, and a reduction in leisure activities. For many of us, our entire self-esteem is wrapped up in one or all of these aspects of our lives. Now, when someone says "What do you do?" you may not respond with "I'm a trucker" or "I am a legal secretary." Instead, you may think to yourself, "I am a failure" or "I sit home all day." When you no longer have an occupation with which to identify, your self-worth may suffer.

Being with friends and doing for them and your family may have been your identity. Instead of being able to take an entire meal over to a sick friend or drive your neighbor to have his car fixed, you are the one who needs help. If you have been a very independent individual, this switch to dependency has probably taken its toll on your self-esteem.

Survival Strategies for Combating Low Self-Esteem

1. Take your focus off the negative aspects of your life.

2. Make a list of all your good qualities.

3. Remember that your family's love isn't based solely on what you do for them or the role you play in the family.

4. Allow yourself to consider less demanding types of employment that would occupy your time and make you feel worthwhile.

5. Do not avoid social interactions. In the end this only makes things worse.

6. Try to do as many things for yourself as you can. You will feel better the more independent you become.

Coping with Physical Ailments

You know that when you feel bad, your outlook on life takes on a negative dimension, and little obstacles appear to be insurmountable. Although you most likely had aches, pains, and physical ailments before the onset of the chronic pain, you were emotionally capable of handling these minor inconveniences. Now that your energy is expended toward managing chronic pain, however, it is more difficult for you to accept and/or ignore these irritating, but minor, physical problems.

In addition, the specific cause of your chronic pain can ultimately cause other physical problems. For example, you avoid putting pressure on your left leg due to sciatic nerve pain, but this leads to tight muscles in an area that originally was pain free.

Survival Strategies for Avoiding Other Physical Ailments

1. Limit the references you make to your pain in conversations with family members, even though you may be worried.

2. Do not bore your friends with excessive descriptions of your problems. They are probably generally concerned about your pain, but do not want to hear blow-by-blow descriptions of your ongoing difficulties.

3. Visit a physician to discuss any additional problems you may be having. This should help ease your mind. If the doctor says that the other problems are not serious, be satisfied with the diagnosis. (You should always feel comfortable seeking a second opinion.)

4. Consider nonmedical alternatives to pain management such as relaxation techniques, counseling, and biofeedback.

5. Avoid "doctor shopping" to find a physician who will agree with your diagnosis.

6. Consider a physician-approved exercise program so that your body can combat the current pain and avoid "new" pains, as well as increase your tolerance for activities.

You may experience these or other matters in your everyday life, and some may even seem insurmountable. But rest assured that this is not so! *You can exhibit control and win with your chronic pain.* You can make changes in both your thinking and acting. Do not feel you are alone in doing this. There are trained professionals ready to guide you and your family in a positive direction. Ask for help. You will be glad you did.

8

From Patient to Person:
Those Who Are Winning with Chronic Pain

Every day in our clinic we see people who are winning with chronic pain. These patients initially come in for relief of various types of debilitating pain—chronic back pain, arthritis, osteoporosis, nerve pain, and more—that has tormented them for years. Not only do the patients tell of the chronic pain being a burden, but the stories they share of lifestyle changes—including loss of activity, severed relationships with loved ones, and unemployment—are heartbreaking.

But there is hope! These patients are finding relief from their chronic pain and a chance to begin again as they diligently follow the basic treatment program, manage their stress and emotions, and include new treatments for pain relief when necessary.

The following examples represent real case studies of patients who are regaining their lives as they are winning with chronic pain.

WINNING WITH BACK PAIN

Howard S. was seen after five years of back pain. He had been through several evaluations and many medications. He was told that all X-rays, MRI, and other tests were normal. He was frustrated because the pain in his back was constant, he slept poorly at night, and felt sleepy during the work day.

Howard began a regular program of twice daily moist heat (using a whirlpool) and exercises for his back. He tried several noncortisone anti-inflammatory drugs and more than one of the group of antidepressant medications used for back pain.

There was one localized area of tenderness in the lower back which resulted in severe pain when examined. This trigger area was injected locally.

After a few months the back pain gradually improved. Howard was able to be active with little back discomfort. He started playing golf again. He found that the pain control allowed sleep and the day-time drowsiness stopped.

Howard's problem of chronic back pain is actually a common one. There is often constant back pain that gradually limits activity more and more. Tests, including X-rays, may show no abnormalities. This can be frustrating since *the pain is very real.*

The most common sources of back pain in this situation are from soft tissues—muscles, tendons, and other nonbone structures. These types of pain are not signs of serious underlying diseases, but can still result in disabling pain. Trigger areas often contribute to pain in these cases but the exact causes are not known.

Treatment is available once other diseases are eliminated, but it may take weeks or months to see an effect. Patience is needed to find the right combination of medications and exercises for relief.

Tyrone P. is a twenty-three-year-old man who injured his back in a fall at work when he slipped on a wet floor. His pain was severe. After several weeks he had an MRI of the lower back, which was normal, but he continued to have pain so severe that he could not work. His employer offered to change his job but the pain was too intense; it disrupted any activity Tyrone attempted at work. Treatment with moist heat, exercises in physical therapy, and trials with a number of medications gave no relief. Local injections and nerve blocks were also not helpful.

After four months Tyrone was referred to a comprehensive pain clinic. He had inpatient followed by outpatient treatment, consisting of physical therapy, medications, psychological evaluation, and pain control instruction. He performed activities similar to those he would be expected to handle in his job. He returned to work after five weeks, still experiencing some pain, but has not missed any more days of work. He continues an exercise program and medications.

The course of Tyrone's chronic pain is common for those experiencing back pain after a severe injury. Studies show that if there is no improvement and the person cannot return to work after three months, the chances of *ever* returning to work drop dramatically. If medical treatment does not work and surgery is not thought to be needed (a common situation), then referral to a pain clinic should be considered before any additional loss of work occurs.

Some researchers have found that there are specific clues in psychological testing to help predict which persons may be more likely to develop long-term disabling pain. This may allow early detection of those at risk and allow earlier treatment to prevent disability. An effective pain clinic usually can expect about 40 to 60 percent of its clients to return to work, although this can vary with the type of client treated.

Jane W. is a sixty-five-year-old woman who was seen because of pain in the lower back that gradually increased over the course of one year. Even though Jane had noticed some pain and stiffness in her back for years, it had not limited her activities. The more severe back pain occurred when she walked and would stop as soon as she rested. Over a three-month period she noticed that the pain would start after she had walked only one block. Initially she could walk several blocks before the pain began. She was becoming very limited in her shopping and other activities.

X-rays found that Jane had osteoarthritis in the lumbar spine; an MRI showed lumbar stenosis.* There was no improvement in her pain after several months of moist heat, exercises, and medication. In fact, Jane was able to walk even shorter distances before back pain started. She had surgery for the lumbar stenosis and was walking after a few weeks. Six months after the surgery, Jane was walking without any limitation caused by pain.

Richard M. is a fifty-seven-year-old man who had experienced back pain for a year, though he could not recall any major injury. He also had high blood pressure and smoked a pack of cigarettes daily. X-rays of the lower spine showed mild arthritic changes. Richard was found to have an enlargement of the aorta, called aortic aneurism, which is fatal almost 90 percent of the time if enlargement continues and the blood vessel ruptures. This problem can cause back pain as well. He had surgery to repair the aneurism and recovered completely.

Aortic aneurism is especially common in men middle aged and older who have high blood pressure and smoke cigarettes. Internal organ problems can be a cause of back pain and need to be discovered so that proper treatment can be given. In this case, repair of the aneurism was very important, potentially life-saving, and was done in time because Richard *did not ignore his pain.*

---

*In lumbar stenosis there is pressure on nerves in the lower back, as discussed on pp. 33–34.

John T. is a thirty-six-year-old real estate broker who injured his back while playing basketball. After months of pain, evaluation, including a CT scan of the lower back, found a ruptured disc to be the cause of the pain. John tried a medical treatment program including heat, exercises, and medication, a program he followed diligently. However, after several months he could not stand long enough to work a full day. Surgery for removal of the disc was successful, but in the recovery room his heart beat became irregular and then stopped altogether. He was resuscitated and had no permanent ill effects. John has resumed his work without limitations.

John had no medical reasons to suspect that there would be a complication during anesthesia or surgery. He was fortunate that the complication with his heart was quickly and successfully treated. This should remind us to be sure that surgery is performed only when necessary and only after medical treatment has not improved the painful condition. *Also, be sure that the problem being treated with surgery is the one actually causing the pain, not simply an abnormal test result.* Back pain from cancer, for example, would not be helped by surgery for a ruptured disc.

WINNING WITH OSTEOPOROSIS

Helene B. is a seventy-year-old woman who was seen in our clinic for severe back pain. She had noticed a stooped posture over the previous year and had developed severe middle and lower back pain during the past several months. She walked with great discomfort, could not bend over without severe pain, and was fearful that she could no longer be independent in her apartment.

Helene was found to have fractures in her spine from osteoporosis. Her bone density was found to be 50 percent lower than normal (see figure 8.1). She began treatment using moist heat with a warm shower twice daily, slowly increasing exercises for the back, and gradually began walking. She added calcium and vitamin D supplements and Etidronate.

Over a few months Helene's pain subsided significantly. She still had some pain, but experienced no real limitation of her daily activities. After a while, she was able to increase her walking up to one mile each day.

Fractures from osteoporosis do heal, and treatment is especially directed at prevention of the next fracture. Treatment, as outlined on p. 82, is available for osteoporosis.

The heat and exercises help make the back more flexible and limber as well as increase the muscle strength for the support of the spine. Weight-bearing exercises also help strengthen the bones of the spine. The medications used today may help increase the strength of the bones and prevent future fractures. In older persons a main goal is to try to prevent the devastating results of hip fracture, which requires surgery and is frequently accompanied by severe complications (see p. 40).

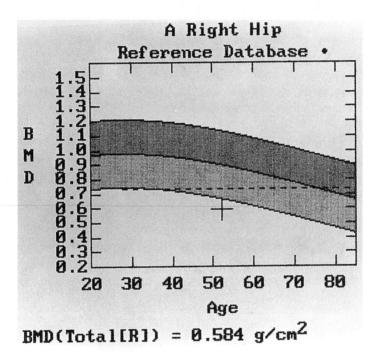

Figure 8.1. **Bone density report shows 58 percent bone loss**

WINNING WITH ARTHRITIS

Lori S. is a sixty-two-year-old woman who has had rheumatoid arthritis for ten years, resulting in pain and swelling in the joints of the hands, shoulders, knees, and feet. She managed her rheumatoid arthritis quite well, controlling the pain with exercises and the medication methotrexate for the arthritis. Lori was very active until she injured her back in an auto accident. She had pain for months and eventually had an MRI of the lower back, which showed a ruptured lumbar disc and lumbar stenosis.

After discussion with her doctors, Lori did not want surgery, so she kept up a program of heat, exercises, and medication. Her back pain is constant and does limit her, especially in walking, but she feels she can live with it if surgery can be avoided. The rheumatoid arthritis continues to be well controlled, with little pain and stiffness in the other joints.

In Lori's case there was more than one problem causing chronic pain. Her rheumatoid arthritis was fairly well controlled by medication, but back pain became much more of a problem. By finding the specific causes of the chronic pain, it became possible to treat each cause separately. In recent years it has been found that the medical treatment of ruptured disc and lumbar stenosis with heat, exercises, and medication can give relief without surgery. Some persons may prefer to avoid the risks of surgery when pain becomes tolerable.

Susan W. is a thirty-four-year-old secretary who has suffered for years with rheumatoid arthritis. For a year she had severe pain and swelling in the joints of the hands, wrists, shoulders, knees, and feet. Susan tried to continue working while seeing to the responsibilities of a single parent, but her pain and fatigue became difficult to tolerate.

Susan began a basic treatment plan for her arthritis, including twice-daily warm showers, exercises for all the joints, and a 15-minute rest period at lunch during work. She began medications for the arthritis, which included methotrexate. After two months she noticed improvement in the pain and stiffness and increased energy. Since then she has gradually improved, and when seen recently she stated that there were no real limits on her activities.

Susan found good treatment for her rheumatoid arthritis, a common cause of chronic pain. The basic treatment of moist heat, exercises, and medication regularly gets results. She has not cured her arthritis (there is no cure as yet), but she certainly has controlled it. Susan has taken care of the pain and stiffness and removed the limitations on her activities.

Dave O. is a sixty-year-old man who has had pain in the left shoulder for three years. At first it was mild but soon became constant and severe. He had trouble lifting his arm to dress and shave, and was limited in his work as a college professor. The muscles around his left shoulder were much smaller and weaker than those on his right side.

Dave had X-rays of the left shoulder, which showed quite advanced osteoarthritis, with narrowing of the joint and spur formation (see figure

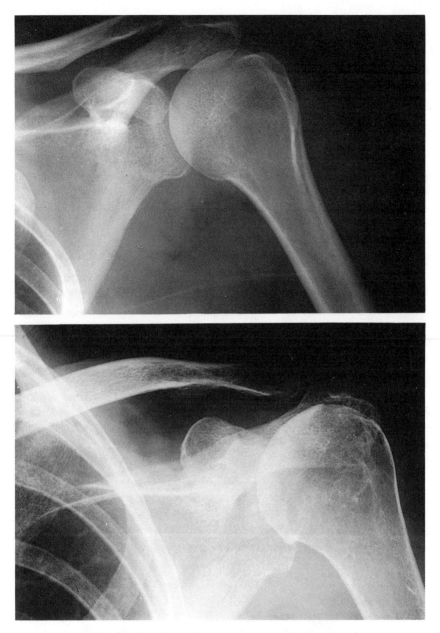

Figure 8.2. Top: X-ray of a normal shoulder
Bottom: X-ray of a shoulder showing advanced osteoarthritis

8.2). He began a regular program of twice-daily warm showers, exercises for the shoulder, and medication using a noncortisone anti-inflammatory drug. After two months the pain was better, and after four months the pain was only mild, with improved strength in the shoulder. Dave felt no real limits in the classroom and was able to perform most other needed activities, using his left arm with no severe pain or discomfort.

Osteoarthritis can affect the shoulder even though no specific injury has occurred. The cause of the arthritis is not known. The pain causes sufferers to use the arm less, which makes the muscles weaker, with even less support for the shoulder. This vicious cycle can actually aggravate the pain and weakness.

A regular exercise program along with medication and moist heat usually brings relief. If the improvement is not enough to control the pain and stiffness, surgery is available in some cases. Most patients improve without surgery, and patients must decide whether the improvement is enough for them. The goal is to be able to do the things you would like to do in reasonable comfort with no side effects from medicines.

WINNING WITH HEADACHES

Jane P. is a sixty-seven-year-old woman who had headaches and neck pain for ten years. The pain was bothersome but she usually either put up with it or took an over-the-counter pain reliever. For several months the pain was much more severe, with headaches constant on both sides of her head. Jane also had worsening of the pain in both jaws when she chewed meat.

After a series of tests, including blood tests and a simple biopsy of a blood vessel under local anesthesia, Jane was found to have temporal arteritis. This is a problem that causes inflammation in the arteries, especially those in the head. It can cause headaches and pain when chewing, and if not treated, can result in permanent loss of vision or even a stroke.

Jane was treated with prednisone, a cortisone derivative. The treatment requires high doses but can be gradually lowered and stopped over months. Her "new" headaches went away, and she was off the prednisone after seven months.

Jane had osteoarthritis with pain in the head and neck for years, but developed a different type of pain that needed new treatment. By recognizing that her headaches had changed, Jane was able to be diagnosed and treated. When your pain changes—when it becomes more severe or seems different—remember that it might be a separate problem that needs its own treatment.

Juanita S. is a twenty-six-year-old woman who works in telemarketing. Her severe headaches started in the back of her head and traveled over the top to the forehead. These headaches caused such terrible pain that Juanita had to leave work early. She did not have the headaches when she was off work during weekends.

After several months Juanita was worried that she might lose her job because she left work so often complaining of headaches. She also thought she might have a brain tumor.

Juanita had a CT brain scan, the results of which were normal and gave her peace of mind. She used a hot shower for the neck and relaxation techniques to decrease her headaches to about one per week. She was eventually able to stop leaving work due to the pain.

These headaches are typical muscle contraction headaches, which often start at the back of the head or neck and may feel like a tight band around the head. These muscles extend over the head to the front of the skull, which is often the path the headache follows.

This type of headaches can be severe and is often related to stress. It may be hard to detect or to admit, but stressful situations often bring on a headache, which can become constant when stress is unremitting.

The treatment can include a pain medication available over the counter such as acetaminophen or ibuprofen. Moist warm towels or a shower can help. Occasionally, muscle relaxants may be needed.

It is important to learn to manage the stress (see chapter 7). This does not necessarily mean quitting your job or leaving the situation. You can actually teach yourself ways to relax the muscles that cause the pain! This can be done by learning biofeedback from a qualified psychologist.

Also, you can teach yourself to perform the relaxation response as shown on pp. 141–43. This may allow you effectively to control the muscle contraction headaches. If the pain does not improve, you should see a psychologist or psychiatrist to learn other ways of effective stress management.

WINNING WITH JAW PAIN

Edith Q., a thirty-five-year-old boutique owner and mother of three, had pain in both jaws for five years. Her activities became more and more limited by the pain, which grew constant even though she had seen many different doctors. Edith had tried many medications and pain preparations without relief. She had even undergone surgery for the jaw pain with replacement of her jaw joints. Yet she continued to have constant jaw pain.

The pain was worse with chewing, so Edith stopped eating and consumed mainly liquids. This diet caused her to lose twenty-five pounds. She also had headaches and neck pain; the nearly constant discomfort made it difficult to work. She often left her job early in the day because of pain.

Edith had gradual improvement with twice-daily moist heat using warm towels and occasionally found relief with ice packs. She began an exercise program twice daily for her neck and back. She gained the most relief from one of the antidepressant group of medications and occasional use of propoxyphene, a narcotic pain reliever. Edith has regained her former weight, and while she still avoids tough and chewy foods, she has resumed her business life with no major limitations.

Chronic pain from the jaws, headaches, and neck pain can be part of the TMJ (Temporomandibular Joint) Syndrome. There is pain from the soft tissues—the muscles, tendons, and ligaments—around the jaws, neck, and head. The pain is often worse with chewing, with clicking sensations in the jaws when opening and closing.

This pain can become disabling. Medications, splints for the mouth at night, surgery, and other treatments are available but there is no excellent treatment as yet. You should be very careful before choosing surgery to treat this problem, and be sure that there is a good chance for improvement in the level of pain. Patience is usually rewarded if a regular program of moist heat, exercises, and trials with available medications is continued, but it may require months before relief begins. In this pain problem, the goal is to make the pain tolerable.

WINNING WITH NECK PAIN

Marlene O., a fifty-year-old woman, suffered with neck pain for ten years after an auto accident. She had a "whiplash" injury at the time and was told that she had arthritis in the neck as a result. In the past two years Marlene had severe neck pain that made her get out of bed at night to try to find relief. Her neck had become weak during recent months when the pain was worse.

Marlene was found to have severe osteoarthritis on X-rays of the cervical spine (neck). Because of the neck muscle weakness, an MRI was ordered. It confirmed the diagnosis. Marlene began twice-daily moist heat using a shower and hot towels. She added exercises for the neck, back, and shoulder muscles. She took several different noncortisone anti-inflammatory drugs until she found one that worked. She also used one of the antidepressant medications (described on p. 76). Marlene showed gradual improvement over six months, and though she still has pain it is tolerable and does not interfere with her activities.

Osteoarthritis in the neck may follow a severe injury and be accompanied by acute pain from the strain of the muscles, tendons, and ligaments. Joints that are injured are more likely to develop osteoarthritis, perhaps because of damage to the cartilage of the joints. This can cause the onset of arthritis at an earlier age than might otherwise occur.

When the pain is severe the neck muscles may become weak. This can mimic other diseases of the spine and spinal cord. The MRI is a good test for making sure there are no ruptured discs, cancer, or other problems that can also cause neck pain and weakness. If other problems are eliminated, the basic treatment plan for osteoarthritis should give relief. Again, the goal is not to cure but to control the arthritis and reduce the pain to tolerable levels.

David R. is fifty-nine years old and has had neck pain for seven years. No injury caused it, and the pain came on gradually. There was a constant low-grade pain in the neck all the time which did not limit David's activities. However, he suffered attacks of more severe pain which lasted days or weeks. These attacks began to occur more often, and were becoming even more frequent and much more debilitating when David was first seen in our clinic. The pain woke him at night and made work as an attorney painful.

X-rays showed mild changes of osteoarthritis in the neck. An MRI of the neck area showed no other specific abnormalities. David began twice-daily moist heat with a shower, and started exercises for the neck and back. Noncortisone anti-inflammatory drugs and an antidepressant drug in low doses brought some improvement, but he still had the severe attacks. During one attack David was found to have a localized trigger area in the upper back which created most of the pain. This trigger point was injected locally. David experienced pain relief the same day. Over months, he had one or two more local injections and continued his other treatment. He now is free of severe pain and has only mild low-grade pain, which does not limit him.

This patient had osteoarthritis in the neck and was also found to have localized areas of tenderness called trigger points in the muscles and tendons. In this case, the severe attacks were solved by local injection of trigger areas and a continued basic treatment plan for the osteoarthritis.

WINNING WITH CANCER PAIN

Estelle A. was a sixty-seven-year-old woman who had breast cancer with surgery and other treatment five years earlier. She developed pain in the back and shoulder. Estelle had osteoarthritis in those areas and the pain was severe and constant. She had bone scan and other tests, which confirmed that the breast cancer had spread to the bones of the back and shoulder.

Estelle was treated by her oncologist but unfortunately the cancer spread to other bones, resulting in more pain. She understood the terminal nature of the illness but wanted to be as comfortable and free of pain as possible.

She was cared for at home with the help of Hospice, an agency that offers home care to terminally ill patients. She was given increasing doses of morphine as the pain became more severe. Estelle was able to be comfortable most of the time, and there were no problems from overdose or addiction over the last six months of her life.

Many patients, nurses, and doctors worry about the problems of addiction or overdose when using strong narcotics for the pain of cancer. Studies show that addiction is actually very unusual in this situation, and the guidelines for standard treatment now include giving adequate doses for pain relief. Other measures are available including nerve blocks, devices for frequent injection of pain medications, and surgery to permanently sever nerves that transmit pain (see p. 140).

WINNING WITH NERVE PAIN

Charles C., a fifty-eight-year-old man, had shingles on his lower back and right leg. The rash broke out suddenly with pain and blisters over his right buttock and down the back of his right leg. The rash went away after a few weeks, but severe leg pain remained. He tried some narcotic tablets his wife had used for cancer pain, but had no relief. After three months of pain Charles entered our clinic.

Charles used several medications, including trials of those in the antidepressant group and the seizure medications. He also used a skin cream (Zostrix) on the painful area. There was gradual improvement over two more months as the level of pain became more acceptable and no longer caused loss of sleep at night.

Shingles (herpes zoster) is an infection caused by the chicken pox virus. It remains in the body for years and can become active again in adults. It causes rash with blisters which usually fade over weeks. Pain from nerve infection can be severe and may last months or years after the rash goes away.

The best treatment is early intervention with acyclovir (Zovirax) to attempt to control the viral infection. Other medications used are from the antidepressant group (p. 76) or from the seizure medications (p. 76). Narcotics do not usually provide very good relief, but some creams have been used with success.

There is no excellent treatment available as yet for this problem, which can cause seemingly unbearable pain. Usually, in time, the pain fades, but it may be only after many months or even years. Your doctor can help guide your treatment, and early intervention is suggested.

9

Between Doctor and Patient:
Questions You May Have

Every day we see people who are suffering from chronic pain. While their symptoms may vary, they all tell of having one thing in common—unending and relentless pain. Perhaps the pain is in the hip or in a shoulder. The pain they describe may be in the jaw or it could be headache pain or pain from a ruptured disc. No matter where the pain is, they all tell of being tired of suffering. Their goal is to live a normal, active life with diminished pain.

Learning from others who have chronic pain is an excellent means of support. Often we can learn a great deal as people describe their symptoms, difficulties, and areas of need. The following questions are the most frequent concerns raised by patients in our clinic. We hope the answers will be beneficial to all who suffer with chronic pain.

BACK PAIN

Q. As a registered nurse in the hospital, I know what pain can do to people. But I never thought it would get the best of me until I tripped going down stairs a few years ago. Since then, I have had severe pain in the lower back. Now every day when I awaken, I have pain. I have difficulty being cheerful and helpful to my patients because my body aches so. I do take my medication, but should I be doing more?

A. Your chronic back pain has definitely changed your life. The first step for you is to get the right answer regarding the cause of the pain. Your doctor can help decide this. There are many possible causes of your back pain, most likely soft tissue pain (pain from the muscles, tendons, and ligaments) from the fall, arthritis such as osteoarthritis from injury, or a ruptured disc in the lower spine. But you still can have any number of other causes of back pain, even those not related to the injury.

Once the cause of the pain is narrowed down as much as possible, then a treatment plan can be created. If there is no cause that can be specifically treated, such as surgery for a ruptured disc, it would be a good idea to begin a program as discussed in chapter 3.

This program for treatment would include the use of moist heat (a warm shower, whirlpool, or bath) for about twenty minutes twice each day.

At the same time, add exercises for the back. Begin with one or two of each back exercise per session, then gradually increase up to five, then ten, and eventually up to twenty repetitions of each exercise twice daily. It is very important to do the exercises regularly.

We suggest that you also begin a very short walk each day, even if only a few yards at first. Then gradually increase the distance. The speed of the walk can be slow. Just make yourself do it every day.

It will take a few weeks to see the effect of the heat and exercises, so do not give up. The longer you do the exercises the greater the chance that you'll build a stronger and more flexible back. This is probably the most critical part of the treatment program.

Medications may also give further relief, with possibilities including one of the noncortisone anti-inflammatory drugs and one of the other group of medications used in the past as antidepressants. Try to remember that there is no good way to predict which of these medications will work for you before you try them. This means you may need to try several different ones before you find the right combination.

Fortunately, most persons do obtain noticeable relief. If you still do not begin to see results after several months, you should talk with your doctor about one of the other available ways to treat the chronic back pain discussed in chapter 5. This could be a good time to go to a pain clinic for evaluation.

Q. What is ankylosing spondylitis? My thirty-year-old brother was just diagnosed with this after suffering with back pain for months. Is there a cure? How did he get this?

A. Ankylosing spondylitis is a type of arthritis more common to men than women and usually begins in adolescence or young adulthood. Many persons have other family members affected also, as discussed on p. 45. There is pain and stiffness in the lower back that persists over months or years. The back pain usually improves with some activity and worsens with prolonged rest and inactivity.

There is often a feeling of stiffness in the morning, and commonly fatigue. About half the time there is arthritis in the shoulders, hips, or other joints. The arthritis may gradually involve the middle and upper back and the neck over five to ten years. Treatment is possible to control the pain and stiffness, and can greatly help prevent deformity.

Prevention of deformity is critical since this can allow continued nearly normal activity, including work and recreation in many cases. Exercises for strengthening and improving posture (discussed in chapter 4) are a major part of the treatment of this type of arthritis.

HEADACHE

Q. No one gets chronic headaches quite like mine. When my head starts to hurt, I know to go and hide in a darkened room. I do not want to see anyone or hear a sound. Lately my headaches have been more frequent, to the point that I am staying at home more and working less. I wonder if I have a brain tumor. I've got to get control of this pain; it is ruining my life, and I'm only twenty-three years old.

A. Headaches can cause chronic pain when they recur repeatedly. It sounds as if your headaches are interfering with your job. First, with severe headaches you should be sure no underlying serious cause is present that can be treated (e.g., hypertension, sinus infection, an abscessed tooth, or other treatable medical problem).

Of course, it's not common but the presence of a brain tumor is a possibility. A brain tumor is actually not commonly the cause of chronic headaches, but it is the cause that may create the most worry. See your doctor. If your headache is severe, your physician will probably recommend a CT scan or MRI test of the head, either of which would find a brain tumor if one is present.

If no other medical problems are found and your headaches are typical of vascular headaches, then there may be medications that can prevent the headaches. There are also medications available, including an injection, that can relieve the acute pain of many vascular headaches such as the migraine, discussed on p. 51.

If muscle contraction headaches are the cause (actually the most common cause), then make a plan to evaluate honestly your own stress levels and how you are managing the stress. Effectively controlling stress may be the best treatment for this type of headache.

Other good treatments for muscle contraction headaches are discussed on p. 96. Relaxation techniques, exercises, and medications are available to control this pain. You can probably find a solution, but it may require trying more than one treatment. As with most types of chronic pain, be determined to continue until you find your answer.

NERVE PAIN

Q. For about three years I have had burning pain in my legs. It is most severe at night and makes me get up out of bed. During the day it is tolerable and actually improves when I walk. I've tried all kinds of pain medicines, but nothing works. Is there anything that can help?

A. The way your pain behaves—the constant, burning pain in the feet and legs that often prevents sleep—suggests that the cause is from nerve pain. The most common type in this situation is called *peripheral neuropathy*—pain from the nerves in the feet and lower legs (see figure 2.13). There are many causes of this type of pain. One such cause is diabetes mellitus, which raises the blood glucose level to an abnormally high level. Treatment here includes control of the blood glucose to as normal as possible.

Other causes of this peripheral neuropathy can be found by your doctor using tests that are usually not complicated. Some cases have an underlying disease that must be treated. Sometimes no definite cause is found.

Even if no specific cause is found, there are medications that often allow control of the pain. You may need to try a few different medications to find the one that works for you, so be patient. It usually requires one to two weeks to be able to tell if one of the medications discussed on p. 106 will give relief.

CANCER PAIN

Q. I am seventy-five years old and have breast cancer. I have had severe pain in the upper back and right shoulder for months, and my doctor told me it was due to the cancer in the bones of the spine and shoulder. Pain pills have given no relief. I can't sleep at night in any position.

A. Cancer pain is especially difficult to tolerate since there is the added worry of whether the cancer itself can be controlled. Your doctor or oncologist (cancer specialist) can best find the exact source of the cancer pain. Often when pain is evaluated in cancer patients a new cause of pain is found. This may be cancer in a new area of bone or nerve.

Radiation therapy may give very good relief of the pain of cancer of the bone. Your doctor can guide you.

When the pain is mild or moderate, nonnarcotic or narcotic pain medications may be successful and used as needed. If the cancer is more advanced and widespread, then higher and more regular doses of narcotics may be needed for relief. A major problem for many doctors, nurses, and patients is fear of narcotic addiction. Research shows that actual addiction by needed doses of narcotics is *very unusual* in cancer patients.

As discussed on p. 139, other ways to give pain relief in cancer include the insertion of a device that allows more frequent injection of medications. This can include injections for nerve blocks to relieve pain. If this technique offers no relief, there are injections and surgery that can cause permanent elimination of the nerve pathways that control pain. With all the methods available most patients should now find it possible to control their pain.

Some newer or less commonly used methods of pain control in cancer are discussed in chapter 5. These methods do give relief in some patients. Many of these can be combined with other forms of pain relief. In cancer pain clinics, all available methods are used to provide comfort in this difficult situation.

JAW PAIN

Q. For weeks I suffered with horrible jaw pain that went into my ears and neck. My physician referred me to my dentist, and after doing a series of X-rays, my dentist told me the pain in my jaw and head stems from TMJ syndrome. What does this mean? He made a splint for me to wear at night when I sleep to protect my teeth. Do I have to wear this for the rest of my life?

A. TMJ (Temporomandibular Joint) syndrome is a type of chronic pain found around the jaw joints (see figure 2.9). It usually includes part of the face and side of the head near the jaw joint. It can happen on the right, the left, or both sides. There may be pain or a cracking sensation in the jaws when chewing. Pain is also felt in the neck and there may be frequent headaches.

There are actually many different causes that can lead to the TMJ syndrome. One cause is thought to be an improper contact of the upper and lower jaws. This produces extra strain on the temporomandibular joints and causes pain in the jaws. This can be made worse by clenching the jaws or grinding movements of the jaws at night. This problem is worse during periods of stress. The splint helps prevent the abnormal forces and grinding and aids in pain control.

The splint is worn at night until there is no pain. Then it can be used as needed. Evaluation of stress and improvement in stress management are also helpful. During periods of more severe jaw pain, soft foods in the diet are suggested. Moist heat or ice packs applied to the TMJ area may help pain control.

Medications that help are those used in other soft tissue pain problems as discussed on p. 99. Be very cautious about having surgery for this problem and make certain you understand what specific improvements you can expect to have. And do not hesitate to have a second opinion to be sure surgery is the best treatment for your own situation.

STRESS AND CHRONIC PAIN

Q. I have noticed that when my life is stressful, so is my back pain. Last week my boss and I had quite an argument over a new client. The next day I ended up in bed with severe back pain. My doctor cannot find the actual cause but rest and moist heat help. Do I need help controlling my stress?

A. There is no question that some people with chronic back pain have much more pain during periods of increased stress. The stress can be emotional—work, family problems, financial difficulties. The stress can even be physical, as in any other medical problem. The exact way in which the added stress creates more pain is not known. The pain is very real, however, just as in any other flare-up of back pain. The stress may not create the back pain, but it does make it worse!

The treatment for these flare-ups resulting from stress is the same as for those from other causes: twice daily moist heat such as warm shower, twice daily exercises for the back, and use of the most effective combination of medications as discussed on pp. 71–72. It may help to add local injection of the trigger area when these are present in the lower back.

Look for ways to quickly reduce stress. Learn the relaxation response on pp. 141–43. This is something you have control over as you learn to deal with stress appropriately. Then as improvement happens, you should take some steps to continue to manage your stress. Stress management may be the key for longer-term control of the flare-ups for your back pain. Taking action as discussed in chapter 7 can begin to control your reaction to everyday stress.

SINUS HEADACHE

Q. Is there any hope for the pain that accompanies a sinus condition? Every time the weather changes, I get horrible pressure in my sinuses and a headache that lasts for days. My nose is stuffy, too. How can I prevent this pain?

A. Chronic headaches from sinus problems are usually treatable. You should check with your doctor. If standard medications do not relieve you, then consider seeing an otolaryngologist (ear, nose, throat specialist) who can find if there are any specific causes in the nose or sinuses. Then if you still have sinus problems, it may be a good idea to see an allergist who can tell if allergies are causing part of your problems.

OSTEOPOROSIS

Q. My grandmother was just diagnosed with osteoporosis. She has a dowager's hump and can barely walk due to pain in her back. Is there anything I can do to help her? She has taken some anti-inflammatory medication, but it has not begun to help yet.

A. Osteoporosis is thinning of the bones, which allows the bones to break more easily. Thirty million Americans are affected. Eventually just the weight of the body can be enough to cause the bones of the spine to compress and fracture. As the bones of the spine become shorter, the person loses height and may become more stooped over. The stooped posture causes a "hump" in the upper part of the back called a dowager's hump because it is found in older women (see figure 9.1).

The fractures in the spine can cause severe pain, especially in the lower spine. But the bones heal, and treatment then is directed toward preventing the *next* fracture. The big danger in osteoporosis (especially

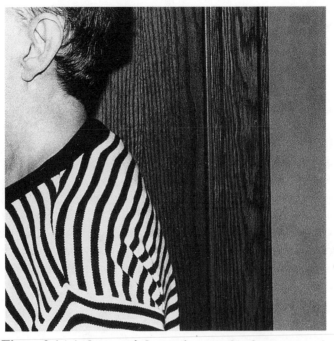

Figure 9.1. A dowager's hump is a result of osteoporosis.

in older women and men) is fracture of the hip, which is often devastating to an older person. It requires an operation to allow walking. Some studies show that up to 20 percent of those affected may die in the first year after a hip fracture.

Anti-inflammatory medications may not help the pain of a fracture in the spine, but the pain usually improves after a few weeks unless more fractures occur. As the pain improves the person can begin to walk, gradually increasing the distance covered. Then an exercise program to strengthen the back muscles should begin to make the back stronger. Medications are available to help increase the bone strength and hopefully prevent future fractures. This is discussed on p. 87.

Since osteoporosis may affect other family members and is more common in women, you should check your risk factors and begin prevention steps. It is now possible to detect osteoporosis early and start more effective medication long before fractures happen.

Q. When I look at my mother and grandmother who both have osteoporosis, I live in fear of getting it. They suffer with repeated fractures and have both become homebound for fear of falling. I am forty-three and quite active, working out at a local gym five days a week. I am also employed as a school teacher and have two daughters. What can I do to avoid the pain they are experiencing?

A. Osteoporosis is a common cause of chronic back pain. The thinning of the bones allows fractures in the spine that can cause severe pain. As time goes on, the spine becomes shorter and more stooped, which can also contribute to the pain.

Unfortunately, most persons find out about osteoporosis only after they suffer a fracture. There are certain risk factors described on pp. 40–43 which make it possible to predict who may be at higher risk for osteoporosis years before any fractures occur. If you have more than two risk factors, then it may be a good idea to ask your doctor if you should have a bone density test (see figure 9.2). This can easily tell if your bones have osteoporosis and can allow treatment. The newer treatments available have a good chance of increasing bone density and hopefully lowering the risk of future fracture, especially hip fracture. In other words, you can probably change what happens years from now by taking a few simple steps today!

PHANTOM PAIN

Q. People think I am crazy, but I have pain where I shouldn't. Let me explain. I am a fifty-year-old male and I had a boating accident. Last year due to some complications, I had to have my right leg amputated below the knee. Now I have constant pain where my leg used to be. Am I crazy?

A. You're not crazy. The pain you're feeling is called "phantom pain" and is very real. Most persons who have had an amputation have sensations that are present in the absent limb. However, some are affected by severe pain in the same area, which may be mild and nonlimiting or severe and disabling.

The cause of phantom limb pain is not known but is thought to be related to the nerve supply to the area of the leg that was amputated. It may fade over months but can last for years.

In those cases of chronic pain, treatment as discussed in chapter 3 is not excellent. Medications such as non-narcotic and even narcotic pain relievers are used, as well as other medications as discussed on p. 65. Other techniques for pain relief are sometimes used, such as TENS

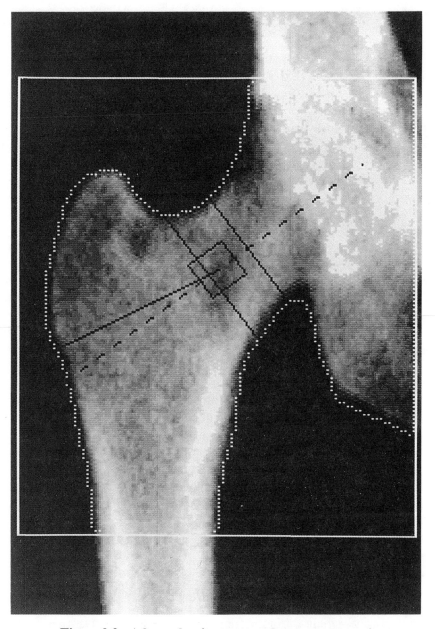

Figure 9.2. A bone density test can detect osteoporosis.

(Transcutaneous Electrical Nerve Stimulation) and at times, surgical procedures are used. If *no* relief is found, a comprehensive pain clinic evaluation as discussed in chapter 3 may be necessary.

HYPNOSIS FOR PAIN

Q. I read in a popular magazine about the use of hypnosis to eliminate pain. Does this really work? If so, how can I find a reputable professional who does this?

A. Hypnosis is another way to attempt to control pain. It is not a new method, but has been used in some novel ways recently. Suggestions are made that allow the patient to decrease the intensity of the pain, to move the pain to another area, or to try to build a feeling of separation from the pain.

Talk with your doctor to find a qualified psychologist or psychiatrist if hypnosis would be worthwhile for you.

TENS FOR PAIN

Q. What is TENS? My grandfather talks about how physicians used this form of pain treatment when he was in college fifty years ago. Now my doctor wants to use this on my back. Can this method still be effective? How does it work to eliminate or relieve pain?

A. TENS is transcutaneous electrical nerve stimulation. It has been used for many types of pain. The theory is that electrical stimulation of certain nerves blocks other nerves that are sending pain signals from the affected area. Another theory is that TENS causes release of endorphins which are a natural form of pain reliever.

The person wears a battery powered stimulator with wires attached leading to electrodes that are attached to the skin with adhesive pads. The electrodes are placed in the area of the pain and the positions of the electrodes moved to find the best relief. A trial of about one month may be needed to decide if this is effective. TENS can be used continuously or only during more severe times of pain. The pain relief may last for a period of time after the stimulator is turned off.

In some persons the trouble of wearing the electrodes and stimulator is not worth the pain relief, but for some it gives good control of pain.

Think of it as one more method of pain control that may be tried if others are not successful.

STRESS AND HEADACHE PAIN

Q. I am not a "stressed" person, but after someone yells at me or disagrees with me, I find that my head throbs. I don't have migraines, and I don't argue back. I try not to react to their anger, but my head certainly does! What can I do?

A. Your headache sounds much like a muscle contraction headache as described on p. 96. If the headaches bother you and are clearly related to periods of disagreement and stress, it would be a good idea to evaluate your stress management. It is quite easy to learn some steps you can take on your own to better manage these times of stress and hopefully eliminate the headache. The relaxation response outlined in chapter 5 is an excellent technique. These steps can be taught by a clinical psychologist experienced in stress management.

LOWER BACK PAIN

Q. I have had back pain for two years since I fell at work and injured my back. Now when I do lifting at work or at home it makes the pain much worse and has caused me to miss more work. I heard recently that a back support that could prevent further back strain and injury could be worn at work or when lifting. Would this help me?

A. There are a number of types of lower back (lumbar) support belts that can be used by those who do regular lifting (figure 9.3). Some workers feel these supports help by reminding them of the correct positions for lifting. Many companies ask their workers to wear these supports or give them the option to do so. They won't prevent injury to the back if you ignore proper lifting techniques. And they can't replace exercise as a very important way to keep the back muscles strong.

Some of the recommendations from the National Institute for Occupational Health and Safety which may help prevent back injury when lifting are:

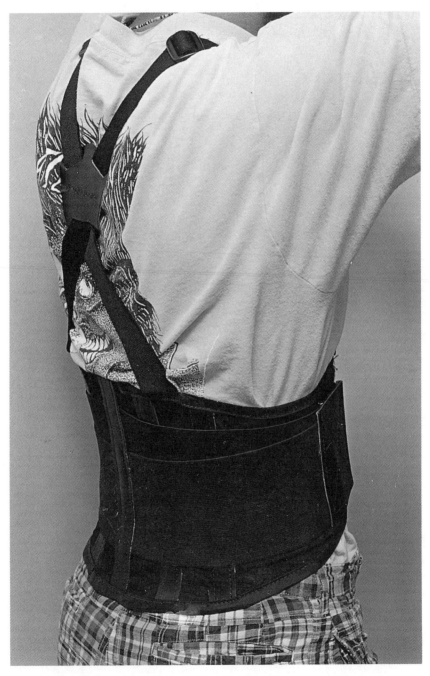

Figure 9.3. A back support can be useful in work situations.

- Try to be about 7 to 8 inches from the center of weight of the object when you lift. Do not hold the object at arm's length.

- Try to lift with your legs, not just your back. This uses the strength of the legs for help in lifting.

- Try not to lift objects higher than the level of your chest. If needed, use a stool.

- Don't twist your body when lifting. Turn your feet if you need to change positions.

- Be sure of proper footing to avoid a sudden slip.

- Get help from co-workers or a machine when the object is too heavy for one person.

HEAT OR ICE?

Q. Which is better for pain relief, moist heat or ice packs? I have had varying opinions from my physicians, and I want to do what is best.

A. For most persons, moist heat helps relieve pain by relaxing the muscles and increasing flexibility. It also seems to have some effect on decreasing inflammation in the soft tissues. The form of heat can vary, but usually moist heat (such as a warm shower, whirlpool or bath tub or hot towels) is more effective than dry heat (like a heating pad). It is used two or more times daily for fifteen to twenty minutes each time.

Some find that ice packs (plastic bags with ice cubes) work as well or better than heat. These can be used for ten to fifteen minutes, two or three times daily for relief. Some persons find ice helps more than heat, especially in acute attacks of pain.

Some find that alternating heat with ice helps more than either remedy alone. One session is used with moist heat and the next with ice.

Every person is different. Find the system that works best for you, and stick with this until you see relief.

PAIN SENSITIVITY

Q. I sometimes feel like a weak person since I have such a low tolerance for pain. I have lived with chronic back pain since I ruptured a disc playing football in college. Since that time I avoid activities with my friends for fear of having mo⁻⁻ pain, and they tell me that I complain too much. Do I just feel pain more than others?

A. This is a good question, because pain is felt by each individual differently. Severe pain for one person may not be so for another. It is not known exactly what causes some people to be more sensitive to pain than others.

It is likely that many factors are involved, including personality. Some people seem to be more stoic than others, and certain people express their feelings more than others. In some cultures it is a sign of weakness to show pain, and young men go through elaborate rituals to demonstrate their ability to tolerate pain without expression.

For each person, the combination of culture, personality, and specific cause of pain is managed differently. In treatment of chronic pain this can be taken into account, but each person's own perception of pain, whether mild or severe, is usually accepted. Treatment is aimed at controlling that person's pain. Personality factors do play an important role and can be used to help control pain as discussed in chapter 7.

RHEUMATOID ARTHRITIS

Q. I have rheumatoid arthritis and have been in pain ever since I can remember. I'd give anything to be able to work in my garden again. What can I do to make this goal?

A. Rheumatoid arthritis, whose cause is unknown, is usually a chronic condition with chronic pain. There is inflammation with pain, swelling and stiffness in the hands, wrists, elbows, shoulders, knees, ankles, feet, or almost any other joint. There can be terrible fatigue, with morning stiffness that may last for hours. Many daily activities, such as working in the garden, can be impossible.

Be sure you have proper diagnosis and make a plan for treatment. This should include a basic program of twice daily moist heat (a shower is good) for ten to twenty minutes. Add exercises for the joints as described in chapter 4, and gradually increase from only one or two up to twenty of each exercise twice daily in the shower or right afterward. This will increase strength and flexibility.

Medications are important in rheumatoid arthritis. One of the non-cortisone anti-inflammatory drugs often gives relief, but you may need to try a number of them, under a doctor's supervision, to find the right one. If there is not enough relief, then one of the groups of drugs that suppress the arthritis at a more basic level is added. These are slow-acting but provide a good chance of excellent control of pain and stiffness with improved activity. You may need to see a rheumatologist (an arthritis specialist).

Your activity can increase as you recover from the pain of arthritis. There are actually very few limits on activity as long as you do the prescribed exercises twice daily and as long as there is no severe pain. We encourage the fullest activity possible. One patient with rheumatoid arthritis who was fishing in a river in Montana was asked why she was there if she had arthritis. She answered that if she had the choice of hurting at home or hurting outside, she would rather be outdoors enjoying her life!

OSTEOARTHRITIS

Q. I don't know which is worse: my ever-present knee pain from osteoarthritis or the anger I feel inside. When I look at my retired friends playing golf or swimming laps in the country club pool, I feel cheated. I stay indoors all day, sitting in my recliner. What can I do? I want to enjoy my life.

A. Osteoarthritis is the most common type of arthritis, caused by wearing away of the cartilage that cushions the joints and makes them move smoothly. If you have become unable to do the things you want to do, you should definitely take action. First, be sure that you are following the basic program of moist heat twice daily and exercises twice a day. Especially important are the exercises described in chapter 4 for the knees, hips, and back since these muscles support the knees.

Medications are available in osteoarthritis. One of the noncortisone anti-inflammatory drugs may give relief—most patients find one, but it may require a period of trying several kinds, under a doctor's supervision, to see which works best. If still not enough relief is obtained, then a local injection of a cortisone derivative into the knee may give temporary relief, and usually lasts from several weeks to a few months.

If you still cannot get around and do the things you would like, including golf, then you may need to see an orthopedic surgeon. This specialist can tell you if a total joint replacement would help your pain.

Be sure that you let the surgeon know what activities you want to be able to pursue following surgery. And don't forget that after surgery the work begins—therapy to make the muscles strong and the joint flexible. Recovery can be easier and faster after surgery if you are already on an exercise program for the arthritis.

BURSITIS PAIN

Q. How do you convince a husband and three teenagers that the pain in my shoulder from bursitis is not, in fact, in my head? They think that I look "perfectly healthy" and expect me to function as usual. But my shoulder aches persistently to the point of tears. Is there any help for me?

A. Chronic pain in the shoulder can be disabling and discouraging, especially when others don't understand your pain. It is very common for many arthritis patients to "look OK" and thus receive little sympathy. The best idea is to realize that even your family may never understand and that you shouldn't expect any sympathy.

You should be certain that the pain in your shoulder is in fact due to bursitis by checking with your doctor. Then be sure you're following the basic treatment program of twice daily moist heat—in this case a warm shower is probably the best—for ten to fifteen minutes. While in the shower, do the shoulder exercises starting with one or two and gradually increasing to twenty of each twice daily. These are shown in chapter 4.

One of the noncortisone anti-inflammatory drugs may offer good relief of pain and stiffness. If not, a local injection of a cortisone derivative often provides good relief safely. This may also allow you to do the exercises more effectively.

If after a few months there is no improvement, it may be a good idea to consult an orthopedic surgeon to see whether there is a tear in the rotator cuff, the group of tendons and other tissues around the shoulder. This or other problems may have other treatments available for relief of the pain. It would be unusual in your situation to have simply to "live" with the shoulder pain.

NECK PAIN

Q. My doctor has recommended that I learn relaxation therapy to help with my chronic neck pain. I have tried medications and exercise, and I feel some relief, but the medications upset my stomach so much that I can hardly take them. My doctor said that with the relaxation therapy, I can probably reduce my medications and still feel relief. Is this true?

A. Neck pain from many causes can be aggravated by tightness in the muscles of the neck and upper back. This can be made worse during periods of stress, with pain extending from the neck over the top of the head like a tight band. Many find that learning to relax the muscles can be more effective than medications for pain relief. The relaxation response is a technique that you can learn to help relax the muscles of the neck and other areas of the body. This can be important because researchers have found that relaxation techniques can reduce anxiety, tension, and stress—and chronic pain is a major source of stress, physically and mentally.

The acute physical pain causes physical stress. And the body's common response is to make muscles tense and more tight. This can actually increase the amount of pain and start a vicious cycle of pain, as well as more muscle tightness. But relaxation (which can be learned) can reduce excess muscle tension and remove the "added pain" that is felt when the muscles are tight and tense.

The stress of chronic pain also adds emotional and mental demands and alters people's moods. The worry of the pain becoming worse may increase the stress even further.

The relaxation response can reduce some of the emotional stress of pain by adding inner quiet, calming of negative thoughts, and a mental focus away from the pain.

You may be able to begin learning the relaxation technique by the steps given on pp. 141–43. It is well worth the effort and also can be taught by a qualified clinical psychologist as discussed on p. 177.

PAIN CLINICS

Q. After living with chronic back pain every day for seven months and trying different medications and forms of treatment, my doctor has suggested that I should go to a pain clinic. What do I look for? How do I know if it is right for me?

A. If the treatment measures outlined in chapter 3 do not provide pain relief and improvement in activity, then it is a good idea to consider evaluation by a pain clinic. There are several types of pain clinics, with emphases on different aspects of pain treatment. Some medical clinics may emphasize medications, injections, and other similar measures. Physical therapy with exercise and conditioning may be featured at other clinics, and psychological evaluation and treatment at still others. The emphasis in a pain clinic is usually determined by the interests and experience of its staff.

Comprehensive pain clinics, on the other hand, combine all available methods for evaluation and treatment of pain. The cost is higher, but if it controls pain and allows you to return to work, it will be well worth the expense. Forty to sixty percent of patients may return to work after this type of treatment.

Your doctor can help you choose the clinic to consider if the methods tried at home or in the doctor's office don't give relief. The specific areas a pain clinic needs to address are:

- relief of chronic pain

- increase in activity

- success in returning to work

- lower use of medication

- less need for medical care.

A comprehensive clinic should have a wide variety of help from physicians, nurses, physical therapists, psychologists, vocational rehabilitation specialists, and others. Physical therapy, psychological evaluation and counseling, use of medication and injection for pain, stress management and followup can all be implemented at a reputable pain clinic (see chapter 3 for more information on comprehensive pain clinics).